Your Health Creation

Dr Matous Bursik

This is an IndieMosh book

brought to you by MoshPit Publishing
an imprint of Mosher's Business Support Pty Ltd

PO Box 147
Hazelbrook NSW 2779

indiemosh.com.au

Cataloguing-in-Publication entry is available from the National Library of Australia: http://catalogue.nla.gov.au/

Title:	Your Health Creation: Your Health Your Way
Author:	Bursik, Matous (1977–)
ISBNs:	978-1-925666-46-5 (paperback)
	978-1-925666-37-3 (hardback)
	978-1-925666-19-9 (ebook – epub)
	978-1-925666-20-5 (ebook – mobi)

Front cover design by Lee Hutchinson

Cover layout by Ally Mosher

Contents

Introduction

Start of a Journey

"Health is not a destination, it's a journey"

~ Unknown

If you have picked up this book it means you are interested in the way health operates in yourself and in the world. In fact, this book was written to answer a few simple questions about the nature of life. Answers that hold a key, that can unlock the doors that lead to our dreams, and enable us to create a life of value.

The questions of inquiry are simply:

— *What is health and how does life create it?*

— *How can we create it in our own experience?*

At first, when I sought the answers this inquest presented, they seemed quite ordinary. It seemed that way because, like many people, I took my health for granted. It was only when I lost it for a while, that its value became profoundly illuminated. As I journeyed towards the answers, I realized that the journey itself contained a hidden treasure, that has the potential to heal the world.

My Health Creation Journey Begins

Reflecting on my life, I have been on a journey to answer these questions for far longer than I have been aware. It was my journey that became my greatest teacher, and has made me realise that health is not a destination, but rather a way of seeing the world. The way we choose to create ourselves, as we walk through the circumstances of our lives. Because of this understanding, I can appreciate the peaks and the valleys, and all the terrain that has constituted my experience of life thus far.

My interest in health started in childhood. Even though I did not think of it in that way before, I had a keen curiosity about life, how it worked, and its innate purpose.

In high school, this curiosity led me to focus my studies on science, exploring physics and chemistry, trying to understand the laws that govern life. But knowing was not enough. A part of me wanted to experience it first-hand. This led me to explore the arts. Playing musical instruments, acting, and singing brought a level of experience to life that knowing simply could not. However, I chose to pursue my studies in science at university because I wanted to understand—not only for myself—but in a manner which I could share with others.

Living things became my interest and I began to study biomedical science. Life brought an added dimension which sparked new possibilities. Although stars and objects always seemed to follow set laws that you could write in an equation, people and animals did not. There was an element of free will that made the whole experience unpredictable and mysterious. This mystery whispered to my heart and set the compass for my journey.

My desire to know and understand health was driven by curiosity, but as I grew and learned more about the world, it became equally driven by the expressions of suffering and dysfunction of the human experience that I witnessed.

Studying the history of humanity and traveling the planet in my early twenties, I realized that humans found it difficult to live in this world in a healthy manner; from unspeakably cruel and brutal wars that litter historic writings, to social discord that led to the expression of many preventable diseases, the suppression of women's rights, racism, and an unreasonable gap between rich and poor, which drove the creation of poverty.

Yet humans have not only created conflict with ourselves, we are also destroying the natural ecosystems, upon which all of life depends, as we strive to become bigger and better. Through unchecked population growth of the human species, the environmental destitution of the world's rainforests, and ever increasing pollution problems: we are destroying the health of nature itself and creating a mass extinction of animal species that has not been seen since the last Ice Age. It is as if, even though the human species placed itself at the pinnacle of intellect and knowledge, somehow we forgot—or perhaps never learned—how to live in a healthy manner with each other and with our environment. Even now we are altering the climate of the whole planet.

Quite literally, our planet has a fever. It is not well.

Surely there must be an answer to these seemingly insurmountable problems?

Pondering these problems and conflicts motivated me to try and make a difference in the world. As I finished studying science I applied for medicine at the University of Sydney, Australia. Perhaps in this profession I could make a small difference. Learning about illness in people might help me discover how best to find solutions to create health. Yet for some strange reason, my studies did not take me to where I wanted to go. The course focused on the hundreds of disease processes inflicting human beings. But why life operated like it did, and how health was created hardly seemed to come up. We became so busy in understanding and fixing or trying to prevent a vast array of illnesses, that we simply had no time to ask ourselves what actually constitutes health in the first place.

It was as if there was something missing. It was as if the whole medical system was broken into a hundred pieces. Specialists study for a decade to understand each piece and how it could be repaired when broken. Yet the understanding of how it all came together, in a healthy manner, was difficult to grasp with a mind of reason—and rarely entertained.

Perhaps the answers could be found elsewhere?

I turned my attention in my spare time towards philosophy and religion whose main purposes seemed to be bringing meaning to it all. There I found many interesting ideas and perspectives on life. Yet having been trained in science and medicine, with logical and technical thought, I found the philosophies were so often lacking in practical application when compared to the science I was studying at university. There was a great chasm between the two worlds. It made me wonder if somehow their realities could be bridged.

Beyond my curiosity or seeming altruism to solve the problems of the world, there was a personal crisis I was trying to address, driven by conflict in my own world. Although I have always been lucky in my physical health, I could see the same conflicts and problems society was experiencing in relationship to the world were echoing in my interpersonal relationships. I was like a microcosm of the great macrocosm. I simply did not understand why.

The more I tried to fix it, the more the answer eluded me and the same problems arose time and time again.

I had reached the end of the road paved for me by others, and had not found what I was looking for. But it was here, at a point in my life where internal conflicts were causing havoc in my personal and professional life, that I decided to make a stand and stop looking for answers in books, philosophies, science, or advice. I started my journey inwards. But this time, I decided to stop looking to solve my problems and instead start with the solution. This is where my journey towards health reached conscious awareness.

> — *What is health?*
> — *How can I understand it?*
> — *How can I experience it in my own reality?*

At this point of my journey I had an epiphany—an insight into the nature of life. Something inside of me opened my awareness to a field of consciousness that animated life. It was an experience so meaningful and so powerful that it changed me fundamentally.

Vitality—My Experience of Health

It took me several years to fully understand, integrate, and translate my experience into words and concepts that I could understand with my logical mind. Much of it seemed so different to what I had been taught.

What I discovered is that within us there resides a field of awareness, which I call "Vitality", forming the framework of healthy expression in living things. My journey to understanding its dynamics became the inspiration for this book. For Vitality was the foundation that enabled health to exist in living things. In essence:

Vitality is health flowing through matter.

The journey was not easy. Looking deep within often challenges the fabric of one's understandings and reality. It takes courage. In a way I was on a mythological journey of growth and understanding. I faced my deepest fears, experienced my greatest failures, and almost destroyed all that I had worked hard to create, trying to see through my own misperceptions of the world that I did not fully understand. Yet, as with any mythological journey, it is these trials and tribulations, failures and learning cycles that enable us to find clarity and deeper meaning. It is to grow in understanding of one's own reality.

Looking back now, I am grateful for all of the difficulties, for they have led me to where I am today.

Health Creation

I have been a medical doctor for over a decade, focusing my work on emergency medicine. I have studied the ways illness and disease operate, such that we can diagnose them and then intervene to fix or heal and restore health. Yet now I looked at my world upside down asking:

— *What if we could **start** with health?*
— *What if we could understand its dynamics and seek to create it in our lives?*
— *Would this not increase our chances of keeping it in our reality?*

This idea excited me. After all, health is the secret ingredient of life that makes all things possible. Health is the foundation upon which life itself stands.

Why Health?

*"It is health that is real wealth, and not pieces of
gold and silver."*

~ Mahatma Gandhi

Considering the nature of health is important because it is the foundation on which life takes place. With health, a person is given the opportunity to live life to its full potential, to engage in physical activity, to think and feel freely, to relate with and contribute to society in a meaningful manner, to enjoy interpersonal relationships, and seek happiness and deeper meaning within the context of their own lives. At its peak, health has the power to transcend conflict and fuel creativity, meaning, and love in one's life.

Health is the platform on which our lives are built. Therefore, it is perhaps our greatest asset, for it unlocks all other gifts that life bestows upon us.

Put another way, if life was a gift that gave you a million pieces of value, then health would represent the "1" at the start of that 1,000,000. Although "1" does not seem like much when compared to a million, when it is present, we can add as many zeros behind it to create a life of increasing value and worth. However, when the "1" is absent, all the zeros in the world come to naught. In a very real way health is not only the foundation of our wealth—it *is* the wealth we are looking for.

Despite its value however, health is often taken for granted. It's only when illness takes hold that we start to focus on what has gone wrong. Our whole health care system in the Western world has been developed around answering these questions:

— *What is illness?*
— *How can we fix it?*
— *How can we prevent it?*

Although these questions are very important and have led to the development of a sophisticated and expansive health care system that has enabled us to fix or treat many ailments, I believe of equal importance is the question:

— *What is health?*

Only in understanding the answer to this question can humanity start to undertake a journey that will enable us to create health in our reality, and maximize our chances of keeping it a part of our experience throughout our lives. Not only health in our bodies, but also health in our minds. This health ripples out and impacts the way we relate to other people and our environment, to the way we construct our society. In essence, health has the power to ripple outwards and create itself in the world at large.

Vitality is Our Nature

Your Health Creation reflects my own journey and translates the experience of what I term "Vitality" into a logical understanding. I hope that as you walk with me through its pages you find insight that aids you in creating health in your experience and freedom to live your life in *Vital Abundance*.

This book is founded on a vision of worldwide health. It hopes to enable people to understand health in its totality, so they can create it and experience it in their reality.

Yet as we journey to the understanding of health, we will realize we are simply seeking the essence of who we are. Deep down below the surface of our conscious minds, below the scripting of ideologies and belief systems, resides the ocean of Vitality itself. After all, we are alive, and Vitality is already present in us, waiting for us to embrace its flow. Because we are alive, our bodies and minds are able to access the innate wisdom that creates health. Therefore, creating health within the context of ourselves and our society—and our world at large—is not only our destination, but our destiny.

For we seek, that which we already possess.
We are the magic which we have been seeking.

So let's begin our journey through Your Health Creation, and begin to unlock its mysterious dynamics.

Chapter 1

Your Health Creation

"The whole is greater than the sum of its parts."

~ Aristotle

The Parable of the Elephant

Once upon a time, many scholars, people of government, and religious leaders gathered to discuss the nature of life. There were arguments between them ranging across a vast array of topics. After much quarreling, they finally decided to seek the advice of a female elder who was known to hold much wisdom. She told them a story:

> *Once upon a time there was a King who called to his servant and said, "Go and gather together in one place all the men of this city who were born blind." The servant went forth, and the blind men were assembled.*
>
> *"Here is an elephant," the King told the blind men. "Tell me, what sort of thing is an elephant?"*
>
> *The blind men went forward and felt the elephant, after which they were asked to give their answer.*

> *"Sire," answered the first blind man who had felt the elephant's head. "An elephant is like a pot!"*
>
> *"No, an elephant is like a winnowing basket," said the man who felt the ear.*
>
> *"I think the elephant is like a rope," spoke the man who felt the tail.*
>
> *"Nay, it is like a strong pillar," cried the man who felt the leg.*
>
> *"I think it is like a mortar," said the man who felt the back.*
>
> *And as each opinion was given, the men began to quarrel, each defending their position, trying to explain why the elephant was the way they felt it to be …*

The wise woman paused, then spoke her wisdom:

> *Many cling and wrangle to their perception of life.*
>
> *Yet they only see one side of things, and are blind to the reality of life.*
>
> *~ Indian Parable*

The Question

What is health? Where does it come from?

The answers to these questions lie at the heart of this book. When we think about health we have to take into consideration many elements that span a vast array of fields. We have to be mindful of the physical structures that make up our bodies; biochemical compositions that our bodies rely on to function effectively; physiological processes that ensure our cells are supplied with constant oxygen; and energy they require to carry out their purpose.

We have to dive deep into the intelligence that makes healthy expression possible in these physical structures, all the way to the most subtle energetic fields that govern life.

Indeed, when one looks at the human being, the complexity of who we are is quite remarkable. The fact that health prevails most of the time in such a complex living structure is a small miracle that goes unnoticed by most people most of the time.

Yet what is it that lies at the heart of this mystery? How does life take such a complex structure, such as the human body, or even a grander structure like our society and the natural environment, and unify it, such that health is made manifest? This book will take you on a journey to answer this very question.

Let Us Start at the End

Let's start by defining the essence of *what* health is to set the foundation for the exploration of the underlying dynamics that create health within living systems. Piece by piece we shall unravel the secrets of this great mystery so that by the end we can bring all the pieces together—to open our eyes so we can "see" the whole elephant and realize the whole created is far greater than the sum of its parts.

Health: The Sacred Chord

*"When the lost chord is discovered by humankind,
the discord in the world will be healed and the
symphony of the universe will come into complete
harmony with itself."*

~ P.J. Curtis

The word "health" derives from the old English word, *healp*, meaning "whole". Yet life, as we know, is made of a great many parts. Our own bodies are made up of many different pieces. We live as individuals in a world full of unique living species and a myriad of things. Our psyche is a vast arena of ideas, emotions, and thoughts. It stands to reason that health makes whole the many different elements of life that otherwise appear separate. Yet how does life accomplish such a feat? As it turns out, there are three keys, that when played together, enables living organisms to create health in their experience.

The Three Keys

MEANING is the first key to health

Every healthy living organism has an innate meaning created from it being what it is. This meaning is then expressed as its unique purpose. A healthy element of life has a purpose that serves life. As it grows and evolves its purpose may change and expand, which we call its evolution, yet in healthy organisms, meaning is never lost.

BALANCE is the second key to health

Life only functions within a narrow band of existence, suspended in a continuum of perceived polarity. For health to prevail, life honors this balance, always returning to the magical point that unlocks its ability to function most effectively. As we shall discover, living organisms balance a great many polar elements—both physical and psychological—in their quest to create health in their experience.

HARMONY is the third key to health

Health exists within the grace of harmonious relationships. All healthy living elements relate with every other individual element in a synchronous and harmonious manner. This interdependence of life is the hallmark of a healthy living system. As such, living beings are a colorful tapestry of interdependent strands, which together create a magnificent mosaic called "life".

Life is free to create and evolve itself in any manner, as long as meaning, balance, and harmony is maintained.

And there it is. We have only traveled a short distance on our journey to discover the dynamics of health, and already we can capture WHAT health is within a single statement.

> *Health is created when independent living elements, with unique **meaning**, express their individual purpose, and become **balanced** with themselves and their environment. These individuations then relate to each other in a **harmonious** manner, such that they unite to form a unified whole that is greater than the sum of its parts.*

This statement captures the Three Keys that are always expressed in healthy living things, and which create the foundation of health itself.

Yet what does this mean? How do these ideas relate to us? How do they express themselves in us, and in the world at large? How can we use them to construct a healthy life?

In order to answer these questions we have to embark on a journey. We have to journey inside ourselves and discover who we need to become in order to express the keys that govern health in our own lives. It is my hope that the journey through your health creation will awaken the innate knowledge of health residing within us all, so that you may translate the knowledge of health into your own experience.

This point—where knowledge of health becomes experience—changes us, and gives us a great gift, for it enables us to see who it is we are, and how we belong. It is at this point we experience *Vitality*. I call this point the Illumination of Health in our own experience.

Health: Act of Creation

*"If we are creating ourselves all the time, then it is
never too late to begin creating the bodies we want
instead of the ones we mistakenly assume we are
stuck with."*

~ Deepak Chopra

Now that we have discovered the Three Keys that create
health within living things, we can ask the questions:

— *Who is doing the creating?*
— *Where does the expression of health take place?*

The First Creation

When we consider the human being, the most basic
creation takes place at the level of the cells.

Cells are considered the basic units of life, which co-
exist to co-create organ systems that in turn create the
body of a living organism. The intelligence that enables
such creation is encoded in DNA, which in humans,
consists of nine billion bits of information holding the
structural and functional blueprints of the human body.
This information is stored in the nucleus of every cell like
a library. The DNA is copied, decoded, and translated into
a physical expression. The DNA can also be passed on,
generation to generation, as cells divide. The division of
cells takes place many times during an individual's life,
creating opportunity for the evolution of their coding.

In order to create health, cells have to organize
themselves into organ systems, which express different

sets of unique purpose. They have to relate to each other in a harmonious manner, and create the human body that balances the various elements it requires to function in a healthy manner.

The body becomes the expression of health in the physical reality.

The Second Creation

The second creation pathway is that of our psyche. After all, we experience ourselves to be a unified human being. It is our mind that enables this unification to take place.

As an individual unit of life, living in the vast world of living things, our intelligence defines how we relate to the world. As such, our beliefs, thoughts, and emotions have a great impact on our health.

For our lifestyle to be healthy, we have to find our meaning, and express our purpose in our lives. We have to understand how to find balance with the psychological and environmental forces we relate to, and how to create our life in a harmonious manner as we relate to our environment, other living things, and the world at large.

Our lives, now become the expression of health in the human experience.

The Third Creation

From our cells and minds, health ripples outwards creating our environment. For humans, we call this our society, which has the power to affect our health. Yet this is only a small part of a larger picture.

Humans are but one living species on a planet filled with a myriad of life forms. When seen as a whole, planet Earth is a collection of living life forms interacting with each other creating a unified ecosystem. The natural environment itself becomes an influence on our health as a humanity and as individuals.

Human societies, and the natural environment become the expressions of planet Earth.

The Hidden Creator

Although creation is taking place on the level of the cells, our minds and the environment, there is a hidden creator that makes healthy expression in these systems possible.

It is a field of life, that carries within it the intelligence of health which has the power to move living things to organise themselves in a healthy manner. I call this field VITALITY. It is hidden because it is not seen directly, yet its effects echo in all of creation.

Vitality moves billions of cells to co-create themselves in meaningful, balanced and harmonious ways to create a unified whole that expresses itself as a healthy human body.

Vitality moves our minds to express ourselves in meaningful, balanced and harmonious ways to create a healthy life in our own experience that is unified within the context of our physical, social and environmental relationships.

The myriad of living things in our world are moved by Vitality, to come together to create healthy ecosystems. An environment that is founded on the same keys as are used by our cells and our minds, to express itself as a healthy living planet.

The nature of health does not change. It is the same on the level of the cells as it is on the level of the planet Earth. Just like cells have to be "in tune" with Vitality to create a healthy body, humans have to be "in tune" with the same Vitality to create a healthy lifestyle, and all living things have to be "in tune" with Vitality to create a healthy planet. Vitality is the hidden creator that life "tunes" into to make health a reality.

The Vital Flow of Health: The Elephant Lives

"Those who flow as life flows know they need no other force."

~ Lao Tzu

We have discovered the founding keys that create healthy expressions in living things. Cells use these keys to create a healthy body, and the mind uses them to create a healthy social structure and environment. Yet what brings all of this together is the flow of Vitality as it moves through living things.

Vitality is not a static reality. It is dynamic. In a very real sense, it is alive.

The "elephant" is not a statue that stands in the corner. Rather, it is a dynamic process that flows through space and time in an endless cycle of renewal. As such, health is not constructed as a finished product that we can stand back and say, "There, it is done". Instead, it is created as a movement of change. It is an ongoing dance that never ceases in its evolution.

Vitality flows to unite intelligence, energy, and matter so as to animate life in a healthy manner.

Humans have the capacity to feel this field flowing through us when we "tune" into its reality. Connecting to this awareness—with both our bodies and minds—enables us to understand and embody health as an expression in our life. The awareness of Vitality within us is the awakening of the innate knowledge that codes health.

The field is intrinsically balanced, filled with great meaning, and expresses deep harmony in its relationships. It is always seeking to lead the body and mind towards its own reflection, creating healthy environmental expressions. In a sense, it can be called our soul, which never takes its eye off the mystery that creates health in living organisms.

Before we discuss the "Intelligence of Health" that create the foundations for Vitality, we have to address a glaring question that needs to be answered:

> — *If health lies at the heart of living things, if it's our natural state of existence, then where does disease come from?*

Let us start here. Let us first look into the nature of disease, for the understanding of illness will illuminate our understanding of health.

For when we understand something deeply, it no longer controls us. It allows us to change and leave it behind.

Chapter Summary:

1) Health is a unified concept—it unifies individual living elements to create a whole that is greater than the sum of its parts.

2) Health is the platform upon which life takes place. As such, it opens the door to living a life of value.

3) Health is founded on Three Keys: **Meaning**, **Balance**, and **Harmony**

4) The Keys of Health can be understood and embodied in our own lives.

5) Creation of health takes place on a cellular level, that creates our bodies. The level of the mind, that's used to creates our lives, which as a collective ripples out to create healthy social structures and the ecosystems of the world.

6) There is an underlying field of life, I term "Vitality", which holds the "Intelligence of Health." It is the hidden creator that unifies all individual elements of life so that they relate and create themselves in a healthy manner.

7) Tuning into the field of Vitality enables us to express health in the physical and psychological aspects of ourselves.

8) Understanding illness helps us to leave it behind and choose health.

Chapter 2

Manifestation of Illness: Loss of Health in Living Organisms

"Disease is an expression of who we are not."

This book is not focused on illness or disease, yet it becomes a glaring curiosity when one tries to discuss the nature of health. As such, let's take a brief look at the essence of disease to further illuminate the nature of health.

I will not talk about the physical and biochemical mechanisms that describe the disease process—like is common in the Western medical paradigm. Instead, let's discuss the underlying mythological expressions that underpin its existence. In essence, it's the intelligence—or lack thereof—in living organisms that enables disease to manifest in their physical and metaphysical forms.

Health is an intelligent process that manifests itself in living organisms. When living organisms embody this "intelligence" they create meaningful, balanced, and harmonious physical expressions that unify living organisms. This is how health is expressed in our bodies, in our minds, and in the world at large. We can say that when a living individual approaches a balanced position in their relationships, they enter a door that reveals their inherent meaning, which can be expressed as their unique purpose. This enables them to step into a space that is creative and allows them to express themselves in harmonious ways in their relationships to other living organisms and their environment. As a result, there is a unification that occurs, and health is created.

From a mythological perspective, the foundations of illness are created when the "Intelligence of Health" is eroded. It manifests in cellular, psychological, and environmental ways when one or more of the Three Keys to health disappear. When this occurs, the balance point is lost, meaning becomes obscured, and is replaced by a dualistic, black-and-white reality, which finds its meaning through conflict. The "door" to creativity and harmonious relationships closes and harmony cannot be created.

Disease manifests as the unity of life falls to pieces.

It is interesting to note that all physical ailments that occur in the body, such as infection, cancer, and autoimmune disease processes, can be seen as an absence of meaning, balance, and harmony within the physical structure of living organisms. This also holds true for the unhealthy expression in our psyche, such as depression, addictions, and in our social interaction through poverty, racial and gender inequality, and domestic violence, all the way through to the creation of war.

The great global challenges of our time—from human induced global warming to the destruction of natural ecosystems—can be seen as a loss of health on the global environmental level.

The mythological expressions of disease are the same on the microscopic and the macroscopic levels.

In a way, disease is simply the loss of "Vitality" flowing through living matter. It is the inability to unify individual units of life in a healthy manner. In the next couple of sections we will take a closer look at how this happens, by examining some common examples.

Loss of Physical Health

*"Take care of your body—it's the only place you
have to live."*

~ Unknown

When the Keys of Health are lost in the physical body, illness is made manifest. Let us look at some common examples of disease in the physical body to appreciate how this occurs.

Viral, Bacterial, and Fungal Infections: Loss of Harmony

*"Harmony makes small things grow.
Lack of it makes great things decay."*

~ Sallust

Infections, in all their forms, result from the inability of pathogenic microorganisms, such as bacteria, viruses, and fungi, to harmonize with their environment or other living units of life. Instead of expressing a unique meaning that benefits life, their meaning becomes one of conflict. In the human body they multiply and seek to destroy body cells in the process, furthering their desire to dominate the environment and resources of the body.

If left unchallenged, pathogenic microbes cause infection, which can manifest in all parts of the body, and cause illness—or if severe, even death—of the physical body as a whole. Because of the interconnected nature of life, the death of the host often leads to their demise.

It is interesting to note that not all microorganisms are unhealthy. There are many bacteria in our gastrointestinal system that have the capacity to relate to the body in ways that are mutually beneficial. As such, they create harmony in relation to their environment and health prevails. Both they, and the body cells, co-exist in a healthy manner. This means it is not microorganisms that are the cause of illness. It is only when they lack the "intelligence" to enact the Keys of Health—in this case, the key of Harmony—they come to be called pathogens and cause disease in the human body.

Autoimmune Disease: Losing Harmony With Self

"Autoimmune disease—'cause the only thing tough enough to kick my butt is me."

~ Unknown

Under healthy conditions, the immune system is composed of several types of specialized cells whose purpose is to protect the body from unhealthy microorganisms that threaten the health and survival of the body. Once a "threat" is taken care of, these cells revert to a passive state that is in harmony with the body.

Autoimmune disease occurs when our own immune system loses the ability to recognize cells that are healthy.

This lack of "awareness" of vital structures leads to the immune system attacking certain cells of the body that behave in a healthy manner, mistakenly believing they are pathogens that need to be destroyed. This creates conflict and loss of harmony between cellular processes, and manifests as inflammation—the main symptom and hallmark manifestation of autoimmune disease.

There are around eighty different autoimmune diseases. Their symptoms depend on which organ system of the body the immune cells are attacking. Yet the loss of Harmony—a key that is essential for health creation—is the common cause of them all.

Physical Trauma: Loss of Balance

*"It's all in how you arrange the thing …
the careful balance of the design in the motion."*

~ Andrew Wyeth

Traumatic injury is an obvious health problem of the human body, which mostly occurs when we have an accident.

Injuries, such as broken bones, lacerations, and burns are all common presentations to the emergency department. Yet when seen from a mythological perspective (the underlying intelligence that leads to these health problems, which we will look at in the next chapter), they are all caused by a loss of balance in the the body as it relates to three fundamental forces that exist in our world—the physical force, thermal force, and the chemical force.

In order to maintain health, the human body has to strike a unique balance with these three forces, and when this balance is lost, health too is compromised.

Physical Force

When physical force becomes too great, it causes trauma to physical structures leading to bone fractures, skin laceration, or organ injury. However, constant under-exposure to physical force can also be destructive. This can weaken bone and muscle strength over time and lead to osteoporosis (weak bones) and a predisposition to injury. As such, trauma results from loss of balance between the human body and the physical force. This is why exercise, which is balanced to the person's body, is such an important factor in health creation.

Thermal Force

The cells in our bodies are also required to strike a fine balance with the thermal force. They function around a unique balance of temperature, centering around thirty-seven degrees Celsius.

Exposure to substances or environments that are too hot leads to burns. These can happen on the skin, such as being burned by a fire, or more generally to the whole body, such as suffering a heat stroke on a very hot summer day.

Similarly, exposure to low temperatures can be detrimental. When exposed to very low temperatures for prolonged periods of time the body can suffer hypothermia that can lead to frostbite and cellular demise.

Loss of Balance, in the way we relate to thermal temperature, leads to thermal trauma and loss of health.

Chemical Force

Finally, the cellular functions of our organ systems rely on a very fine and sensitive balance in the chemical composition of the blood that nourishes our cells.

The Ph—a measure of how acidic or alkaline something is—needs to stay around a very narrow 7.35–7.45 balance point. Although we have systems in our bodies that ensure this balance point is maintained, even a small deviation from this balance point can affect cellular function, leading to cell demise, which becomes detrimental to our health.

Cellular life can only function between a Ph of 6.8–7.8. When cells are not able to carry out their unique purpose because they have become damaged, or the environment is not balanced, it leads to illness that can quickly become life threatening.

Similarly, the outsides of our bodies, such as the skin and eyes—although much less sensitive—also get damaged by exposure to very acidic or alkali substances that lead to chemical burns and loss of health.

Genetic Disease: Innate Loss of Meaning

"The human genome is a life written in a book where every word has been written before. A story endlessly rehearsed."

~ Johnny Rich

A group of disease processes, which originated mythologically as an innate lack of meaning, are genetic diseases. Genetic disease results when an error occurs in our DNA.

In simple terms, DNA is a sequence of words called "codons", which create the book of life that codes the "blueprint" of the physical body. When several words, or chapters become damaged, destroyed, or are written in error, the cells are unable to read the information and translate it into reality—or do so in an incorrect manner.

The inability to make certain proteins that are essential for certain tasks, or the making of them in ways that are faulty, such that they cannot express their unique purpose, leads to the demise of cell function. So the affected cells cannot express their unique purpose.

This loss of meaningful expression in a cell type, can be passed on to the next generation as cells divide and copy the error, eroding the health of the body. This process leads to what we call genetic diseases.

A specific example of a genetic disease can be seen in a process called cystic fibrosis. In this process, one cell type that encodes a chloride channel becomes damaged, and the cell is unable to create it, it is therefore unable to express its purpose. In this case, the chloride channel's purpose was the regulation of fluid transport across membranes. When damaged, the fluid begins to thicken, creating an environment which predisposes the body to infection in the lungs. Functional problems with the pancreas, and other organ systems of the body relying on this particular chloride channel, are also put at risk.

Disease results as the respective organ systems are unable to carry out their functions in a meaningful manner.

Genetic diseases are many and varied, and affect many different cell types. We know of around 6,000 different types of genetic disease processes. Yet they all result from damage, error—or several errors—in the cell's DNA structure. They lack expression of a certain purpose in the cell, which erodes the ability of the body to create itself in a healthy manner.

Cancer: Loss of Meaning, Balance, and Harmony

"Cancer doesn't respect nothing."

~ David Chase

I have separated meaning, balance, and harmony in my discussion of disease processes, However, in reality—just like health—they are a unified concept that flows through matter and are animated by the field of Vitality. It is really the intelligence of Vitality that is eroded when disease manifests on the physical level. Whether it is meaning, balance, or harmony that is being lost, they affect each other in a direct fashion. The loss of one leads to a loss of them all.

For example, one of the great physical disease processes that is mythologically expressed as a loss of meaning—which then erodes balance and harmony—is cancer. All cancer cells lose their ability to act out their unique purpose in serving the body due to genetic errors in the cancerous cell.

Cancer cells are called benign if they just sit there as a lump, playing no constructive role in the body. We call them malignant if their expression falls further away from health because they lose their ability to keep balanced.

Normal cells balance their numbers through division and apoptosis (programmed cell death). The body, being a limited closed system, knows it can only hold a certain number of cells for health to prevail. Cancer cells multiply in an uncontrolled manner and expand into the territory of other healthy tissues. This means they are not only useless, but destructive to other functioning organ systems. Much like a bacteria, they divide and act in a manner that creates conflict, blind to the fact that they are causing damage that will not only destroy the body, but ultimately themselves, as they are dependent on the body for survival.

This loss of meaning, then balance, leads to a lack of harmony. Conflict, inflammation, and destruction becomes the expression of the cancer, which often metastasizes, or spreads, to many organ systems.

There are as many types of cancer as there are types of cells in the human body. Some are more dangerous and destructive than others. Yet all of them originate mythologically from the lack of meaning, balance, and harmony as they express themselves in the human body. It is a lack of intelligence of health flowing through the physical system: the lack of unified co-creation within living individual cells.

These examples illustrate the way illness manifests when the intelligence of health is lost in the expression of the cells of the body.

Yet cells are not the only aspect of life that flows creative intelligence. The mind—or what can be called the psyche—also has the capacity to flow creative intelligence, or Vitality. It too can lose health when Vitality is lost in its expression. When this occurs, health is lost in the spectrum of our social expression and experience. Let's explore a few examples to get an appreciation of how this occurs.

Social Expression of Illness

"When health is absent, wisdom cannot reveal itself, art cannot manifest, strength cannot fight, wealth becomes useless, and intelligence cannot be applied."

~ Herophilus

Once the Keys of Health become eroded in the mind, the expression flows outwards into our environment and social interactions. It affects the way we experience our lives, the way we experience our relationships, the way we create our social experience. People start to relate to each other and their environment in ways that are unhealthy. These expressions manifest as social problems, which in a very real sense, create illness in our lives, and the body of our society.

Social problems, such as racism, sexism, domestic violence, all the way through to war, originate from the same place. Not only this, their founding mythological reality is the same as that of diseases found in our bodies! The difference is that they are being expressed, not on the level of the cell, but on the level of the psyche as it relates to its macroscopic environment.

What occurs on the level of the mind takes effect on the body of our society.

Let's explore a few common examples.

Displacement from One's Identity: Lack of Meaning

*"When a person can't find a deep sense of meaning,
they distract themselves with pleasure."*

~ Victor Frankl

When people lose their sense of identity—who they are, how they belong, and what they are contributing to society and the world—there is a vacuum created inside them. This vacuum is created by an innate lack of meaning that stalls their creative expression and relationships upon which health depends. When this occurs, the void is often filled with seeking pleasure and aversion to challenging activities. This polarised way of seeing life, leads to an unbalanced lifestyle that creates actions which erode our social health and forms the basis of what we call "social problems".

*Social displacement manifests as the lack of desire
to contribute to society and the world in a
meaningful manner.*

Social displacement leads to apathy towards work or contribution to society, apathy towards caring for oneself and for others. This often leads to antisocial behavior as lack of respect for ourselves and others blinds us to what it means to have a healthy relationship with ourselves and others.

In its healthy state, life requires a natural movement of creation, a kind of dancing relationship with our environment and other people that provides the body and mind with the elements they require for healthy existence. This is fueled by internal meaning that drives and motivates us. When people are disconnected from this natural, creative flow, emotional displacement occurs and social health is eroded.

Sexism: Loss of Gender Balance

"Of all the evils for which man has made himself responsible, none is so degrading, so shocking, or so brutal as his abuse of the better half of humanity: the female sex."

~ Mahatma Gandhi

One great example of a social problem that derives from loss of balance is sexism. This is a loss of balance between the perceived value of genders.

When one looks into history, human society has been struggling with sexism for much of recorded history. Women's rights and values have been eroded, degraded, and suppressed to a large extent for a very long time in many cultures around the world. It is only in recent times that there has been a concerted effort to address this social problem.

Women are starting to close the gender gap, to gain equal opportunity to study freely, to work in any job they desire to work in, to receive equal pay, to vote, and to be elected into leading social positions. Even in Western countries, equality of value of the sexes is yet to be achieved. Yet the problem is more dire than simple inequality.

Studies by the World Health Organization show that thirty percent of women experience physical or sexual violence in relationships. This accounts for millions of women around the world and highlights the great suffering that erosion of health in relationships creates.

Equality does not mean women and men are the same. It's quite evident they are not. Yet balance does not mean sameness. Balance is the ability to assign equal value to feminine and masculine qualities, to value the differences that set the foundation for a creative relationship to form. This balance in value is what creates the foundation for harmony to be created between genders and brings health to this social dynamic. Equality of value also means equality of opportunity, which allows women and men to choose their path in life without being constricted to set gender roles.

When this balance is lost, we see sexism arise.

Instead of relating in a creative way, using the quality of both genders to create life in a meaningful and harmonious manner, society begins to see the gender difference in terms of conflict, which end up being expressed as the mythological "battle of the sexes". This leads to suffering for both males and females, and has led to the violent suppression of women.

Too often men have used violence and suppression to enable them to be seen in a higher and more valuable light, and gain privilege and power in the social arena. In turn, females have used manipulation to counteract the great injustice that has been perpetrated on their gender, causing pain to men. Even though there are great signs that society is coming more into balance with gender, it has been—and in some societies still is—one of the tragic erosions of social health that plagues human societies.

Racism: Loss of Harmony between Cultures

"It is not differences that divide us.
It is our inability to recognize, accept, and celebrate
those differences."

~ Audre Lorde

Racism, like sexism, has been historically a dark shadow on the social landscape. In a healthy social society made up of many cultures, the variety of unique expressions creates a richness of experience. Each culture adds a unique strand of identity to form a vibrant social tapestry. Yet this can only be created if harmony between cultures is maintained. Too often, when we look at the social landscape, and in our recent history, we see the erosion of harmony when it comes to cultural relationships with each other.

There are many examples in recent history of the erosion of harmony in cultural interaction that has led to a loss of social health with devastating consequences. Such examples include racial genocides inflicted in wars of the twentieth century, which saw the brutal killing of Jews in World War II, six million people killed in a space of five years by Nazi Germany, and the tragic death of a million Tutsi by the Hutu race in Rwanda over a one hundred day period in 1994.

These extreme cases are only the tip of a much larger iceberg. In a recent study in Australia—a country which has a successful multicultural society—it was estimated that racism cost Australian society forty-five billion dollars per year due to the psychological disorders, anxiety, stress, and health problems it creates.

The mythological cause of racism is the inability to create harmony between different sets of belief systems.

In healthy organisms the difference is valued, for when used in a creative manner, it has the capacity to add variety and richness to the organism as a whole. This can be seen in cultures that have embraced a multicultural lifestyle. It increases our variety of tastes and experiences. Yet when we forget to value the difference, lose the ability to harmonize, and see difference as an enemy, racism manifests as a deep wound upon the social landscape with the potential to completely destroy the health of the social body.

It is important to remember that health enables creation of a vast variety of social expressions, yet a social group has to be expressing itself in a healthy manner for healthy relationships to be developed. If a social group creates itself in a manner that erodes the Keys of Health, it will become like a pathogen in a body. It declares itself as the only valuable organism and seeks to destroy the healthy expression of the body. Just like the pathogen, it will be stopped by a healthy social body.

Unfortunately creating harmony with societies that engage in highly unhealthy paradigms is very difficult. However, paradigms change and societies evolve from unhealthy to healthy, and that is what humanity is all about. Humans are not pathogens, we are highly intelligent, and have the capacity to change. This is why understanding health becomes a very important key in creating harmony in social expression. Health is universal and it benefits all.

War: Loss of Social Meaning, Balance, and Harmony

*"I hate war as only a soldier who has lived it can,
only as one who has seen its brutality, its futility,
its stupidity."*

~ Dwight D. Eisenhower

When I discussed the complete loss of health in the body, which is the complete collapse of meaning, balance, and harmony, I used cancer to highlight this phenomenon. In the social body, war comes the closest to encapsulate this reality.

Societies go to war because they lose sight of Vitality. They are blinded to how they belong, and their relationship to each other and the whole. They cannot see the balance between their culture and others. Harmonious relationships are eroded and replaced with rhetoric of conflict, blame, anger, and hate that lead to the creation of war.

Although it's easy to always blame another and position oneself on the side of "good", this is an illusion created when living things lose their ability to "see" and experience Vitality in their expression.

When one looks honestly at war and the experiences of people who are caught in its reality, it's easy to see how undesirable, tragic, and utterly devastating this condition is. It's estimated that 160 million people were killed in wars in the 20th century alone. This is more than 4,300 deaths every single day for the 100 year period!

War is a lack of Vitality flowing through the social body and leads to a very unhealthy social interaction. It underlines the importance and value of understanding health and creating our lives along the pathways toward health.

Sometimes deeply unhealthy expressions in our society have to be stopped. Sometimes we have to make a stand. We make a stand because it's what life demands. Yet when we make a stand against disease in the body, the focus is not to blame the disease, but to find a way to cure it.

The healthy society does not see enemies—it simply sees unhealthy expressions.

Would it not be wiser to simply understand life and how it operates?

Health creates life, making it grow and evolve. Helping societies adapt these principles helps to transcend the need for war. This is where the journey is taking us.

Loss of Health: The Entanglement of Body and Mind

"As above, so too below."

~ Hermes Trismegistus

We have seen how the loss of health on a cellular level manifests as disease in the physical body, and how the loss in the psyche manifests as loss of social health. However, we intuitively know the psyche that creates our social reality, and the cellular expressions that create the human body, are not isolated. Like everything in life, there is a connection and relationship between them. There is an entanglement that takes place.

The loss of the Keys of Health in the body flows to affect health in the mind, which in turn influences our social environment. Similarly, the loss of health in our social environment affects the health of the mind, which flows to affect the health in the body. Let's take a brief look at how this occurs.

The cells of the body are not isolated. Their genetics and microscopic cellular processes are only one factor that influences their ability to express themselves in a healthy manner. They are also influenced greatly by the body's environment: the nutrients, minerals, vitamins, and other essential substances that are found in the blood. These nutrients circulate through the body at all times, such that they are made available to all the cells, playing an essential role in the healthy expression of cellular function.

Yet this environment of the body is not isolated either. It is created by the choices we make as individuals. Choices we make with our minds:

— *Where do we choose to live?*
— *What environment do we expose our bodies to?*
— *What do we choose to eat and drink?*
— *How do we interact with our world?*
— *What is the quality of our relationships?*

These are some key questions, and the answers are created by the way we see ourselves, our lives, and the world in which we live. These choices create ripples that affect and sometimes directly create the internal environment our cells are exposed to through our diet, and lifestyle, therefore playing a critical role in cellular health.

Of course, the choices we make are shaped to a large degree by our social situation:

— *What does our society believe?*
— *What is my social circumstance?*
— *What access to resources do I have?*

The statement, "as above, so too below", reflects that the health of the microscopic world is in direct relationship with our macroscopic world. Life is interconnected. There is no separation.

Yet the relationship runs in both directions: if our cells begin to lose healthy expression, say, through genetic error, it is expressed in our bodies. When our bodies lose health, it affects our psyche, and is expressed in the mind.

The mind is a function of the brain that is dependant on the health of the cells that create its structure. As such, cellular disease ripples to have psychological impact. Once our psychological expression becomes unhealthy, and we start to experience psycho-emotional problems, we start to make unhealthy life choices. They then ripple outwards to create unhealthy relationships within the social context of our environment, influencing the whole social order. We can, and do, create an unhealthy society.

Once the identity—or the intelligence of health—is lost on any spectrum of its expression, it affects every other spectrum. Let's look at a few examples.

Depression: Loss of Meaning, Entanglement

"Depression is a common mental disorder. Globally, an estimated 350 million people of all ages suffer from depression. Depression is the leading cause of disability worldwide, and is a major contributor to the overall global burden of disease."

~ World Health Organization

Depression is an example of how loss of meaning can manifest on the level of our cellular reality, our psyche or our environment, and how they influence each other in an entangled manner.

Depression is the most evident loss of meaning on the level of our psyche. It's the inability to see meaning in one's own life, the feeling of being unworthy and disconnected, the inability to find joy in the activities we are involved in. This loss of psychological well-being has a direct affect on the biochemicals that our body produces.

Staying in a depressive state for too long can create an imbalance of the neurotransmitters in the brain, mainly the underproduction of serotonin and dopamine. Making poor choices in the way we consume nutrients also adds to the problem. Yet we can see depression from the other side of the equation: perhaps it is the imbalance of neurotransmitters, as produced by the cells in the brain, that leads to a loss of meaning and a depressed mood.

After all, the mind is a product of the cells that create the brain.

The entanglement becomes even more confusing when we consider that we often feel depressed because of social or environmental circumstances we experience. Perhaps it's the loss of an important relationship, our job, or the experience of physical or emotional abuse. That is the loss of social and environmental well-being driving psychological depression, and which creates changes in our neurochemistry as a result.

Yet the opposite is also true. When we become depressed we often behave in ways that create social circumstances that are not healthy through our actions! Perhaps we neglect ourselves or others, neglect our responsibilities, get fired from our job because we cannot see the point of caring or don't have the energy to work effectively. Perhaps we start to undermine our relationships until it leads to their breakdown.

When meaning is lost, its expression manifests on all levels of the spectrum. Its loss on any level of creation ripples to all others.

Loss of Balance in Nutrition: Entanglement

"Some 795 million people in the world did not have enough food to lead a healthy active life in 2015."

"Around 600 million people are estimated to be obese in the world in 2014."

~ World Health Organization

The imbalance of nutritional substances in our bodies expresses itself in many ways.

To function in a healthy manner, the body needs a unique balance of organic substances: a balanced fuel supply of carbohydrates, proteins and fats to provide the body with energy and the building blocks it uses to develop and repair itself. It needs a balanced supply of essential chemicals, such as potassium, sodium, and magnesium to play key roles in the function of the heart and nervous system. It needs a balanced supply of vitamins, minerals, and essential amino acids, which play key roles in certain functions of cellular processes. In essence, it requires a balanced, healthy diet. If the human body cannot get enough nourishment, then it cannot function properly.

> *We live in a world where we have the resources to provide this balance for everyone.*

It was estimated in a recent study that if we spent just ten percent of what we spend on war—or preparation for war—as a global community on social projects, we would end world poverty. Yet too often, because of unhealthy social structures, we create societies where millions of people go malnourished every year. Examples of diseases from lack of nutrition, such as a lack of vitamins and minerals include: scurvy (lack of vitamin c) or Wernicke's Encephalopathy (lack of vitamin B1). But the most common is simply the lack of adequate food, which leads to malnutrition, starvation, illness, and death. The World Health Organization estimates that 3.1 million children die from malnutrition every year.

Although we observe the loss of health in the physical body on the level of the cells, it's driven by choices we make with our minds. These choices can stem from simply choosing a poor diet that lacks nutritional value, or it can derive from psychological imbalances, such as anorexia, where a person is compelled to starve themselves.

Yet the biggest problem is the way we structure society. We have set up a social circumstance where millions of people in the world live in a state of poverty and simply do not have access to enough food to be able to eat a balanced diet. Not because we don't have the resources to do so as a global community, but because we create our societies in an unbalanced manner that is blind to this key of health.

Interestingly, this imbalance is just as prevalent on the other end of the spectrum—just as much disease is created from overconsumption of nutrients.

Ingestion of too much nutrition is also greatly detrimental to health. Because Balance is a key to health, it becomes evident that more is not always better.

Overconsumption of some substances—that in a balanced proportion are healthy—can lead to toxicity, which harms cells and thus health. An example is Vitamin A. It can lead to eye damage when ingested in excess, yet benefits our vision when taken in a balanced quantity. Yet the most common diseases are caused by overconsumption of fats, carbohydrates, and proteins. This process leads to obesity, which predisposes people to many disease processes, such as Type 2 diabetes and heart disease, which have become an epidemic in the modern Western world.

Although there is a genetic component that plays a role in Type 2 diabetes in some cases, it is mainly driven by unbalanced lifestyle choices: overconsumption of sugars and an under-active lifestyle.

In this disease process, the combination of imbalanced sugar intake and lack of exercise puts increasing pressure on the pancreas, whose job it is to secrete insulin to enable sugars to leave our bloodstream and enter tissues where it is needed. Yet as we overuse the pancreas by over-ingestion of sugars, its capacity to function diminishes. It's like running a horse for too long until it finally cannot run anymore. The pancreas slows down its insulin production, it cannot keep up with the sugar load, and our blood sugar rises.

Over time, a higher concentration of sugar in the bloodstream causes many disease processes to manifest, such as nerve, kidney, and blood vessel damage. The lack of balance in what we consume and how we move leads to disease in our bodies. Type 2 diabetes—along with smoking, heart disease, stroke, and depression—is considered one of the "Big 5" social health problems in Western society, that leads to many health problems. Yet Type 2 diabetes is a symptom of Western culture. Here the entanglement becomes apparent.

One can make a case that our cellular programming, or the way DNA is expressed, leads people to have lifestyles that lead to obesity and overconsumption of nutrients. Yet it's just as valid to blame the way we think and feel, and the choices we make, that lead us to overconsumption.

Of course it can be argued that it is the West's culture of fast food, processed with high sugar content and consumerist culture, that affect our psyche to make poor choices, which then influences our bodies. Several studies show that as countries adopted a Western diet and lifestyle, Type 2 diabetes became more prevalent.

> *Deep down, the loss of balance with our diet*
> *expresses itself on all the levels of the spectrum,*
> *and they in turn, influence each other in a direct*
> *manner.*

Addiction—Loss of Harmony: Entanglement

> *"The opposite of addiction is not sobriety.*
> *The opposite of addiction is connection."*
>
> *~ Johann Hari*

Addiction is now recognized as a very severe disease process that is physical, psychological, and social in nature. Addiction can be seen as an intersection between cellular, psychological, and social expressions, and has a great detrimental effect on our well-being.

Addiction can occur to many things, but drug addiction to chemical substances causes great damage and grief to human beings. Some of the main drug substances include alcohol, cigarettes, cocaine and amphetamines, just to name a few. The United Nations estimates that 200,000 people die from drug abuse every year around the world, and it would cost society 250 billion dollars a year to provide them proper care. When we add the suffering of people who are addicted, and their families, the cost of this illness is truly great.

Mythologically, addiction is created when harmony is lost.

People who become addicted often have poor relationships and experience conflict in their lives, be it social conflict or psychological conflict. The substance of addiction gives a false sense of well-being that momentarily suspends the suffering, the fear, anxiety or conflict they are are experiencing. Yet as the substance's effect wears off, the lack of harmony returns and manifests as a craving to once again end the suffering of a conflicted reality.

Addictive substances only provide a moment of relief, and as their effect wears off there is a need for ever increasing doses of the substance. In a social study by Johann Hari, the cause of addiction was found to be *not the addictive substance* itself, but the *lack of connection* that people were experiencing. The drug was simply a substitute to feel a momentary sense of connection that gave them a sense of relief. Yet when these people were placed in a warm, connected environment, the vast majority stopped being addicted. It was the lack of harmony in their relationships that drove the addiction.

Addiction is an entangled reality. Some people can have "addictive personalities" that are driven by genetic forces and impacts their social reality in an unhealthy manner. Similarly, unhealthy social circumstances that erode harmony can drive people to make the choice to become addicted to substances. This, in turn, acts on their biochemistry and changes their cellular and biochemical reality, making it very difficult to stop the addiction. As such, a psychological problem becomes a physical one. The loss of harmony manifests its expression through addiction on the body, mind and social levels.

Exploring the Causation of Illness: Entanglement of Mind/Body/Society

"There is no causality, there is only identity."

~ David R. Hawkins

We have seen from the previous examples that the loss of meaning, balance, and harmony on the physical, psychological, or social levels affect the other levels in a ripple-like fashion. So the questions that then arise are:

— *What came first? Cellular, psychological, or social loss of health?*
— *What is the primary mythological cause of illness?*

The answer is quite surprising. Even though we often consider the world in terms of cause and effect, health does not work that way. It would be like trying to say that the egg created the chicken, or that the chicken created the egg. Both cases have legitimate logical arguments, yet to resolve this seeming paradox one has to look deeper.

Health, and the lack of it, is created through our identity, not as a result of causation. It is created through who we are. The identity is then expressed on cellular, psychological, and physical realities, which in turn influence each other. To understand health and its loss, one has to look deeper than the level of its expression! We have to look at the level of our character from which the expression is created.

The reason is that life has an underlying unity to it. That is why health is created when seemingly individual parts of life relate to other parts in a harmonious way that creates a whole that is more than the sum of its parts. Even though we consider the body, the mind, and society separate realities, in fact they are not. They too are entangled and connected as a whole. So what happens to one ripples to affect the others. The cause lies at the heart of how the living organism is expressing itself.

In the next chapter we will look at the *mythology* of living things. This mythology forms the basis of who we are, and how we create our identity and determine if our expression is healthy or not. We will discuss the "perceptual realities" that drive the loss of health and the mythology that encapsulates Vitality—the field of life from which health flows. Yet before we do this, let's zoom out and see how the loss of health ripples out to a global level to grasp why understanding its dynamics is so important.

Global Illness: We Live in a Global Village

"If you want to save our world, you must hurry. We don't know how much longer we can withstand the Nothing"

~ The Southern Oracle, in The Never Ending Story

The erosion of the Keys of Health expresses itself in the body and in the social body. Its effects ripple out into the natural world because humans have such a great influence on the natural world. We utilize its resources at ever-increasing rates, and as our societies grow and expand—in such a fast manner in recent history—we cover the whole globe, and encroach and push against the natural environment everywhere we live.

Unfortunately, because humans are often not in tune with how to construct their societies in a healthy manner, it has led to some glaring global problems, which are posing a threat to all the living organisms on the whole planet. The problem is simply a lack of healthy expression that is slowly seeping its reality across the planet.

"How long can our world withstand the Nothing?" Let's take a look at a few examples.

Destruction of Natural Ecosystems: Loss of Meaning, Balance, and Harmony

*"What we are doing to the forests of the world is but
a mirror reflection of
what we are doing to ourselves and to one another."*

~ Chris Maser

The natural environment is the representation of life on our planet. We are simply one of many thousands of living organisms, which together form the body of planet Earth. The planet is sick because we have forgotten who we are. We have forgotten our meaning and purpose. We have forgotten how to relate to the natural environment in a harmonious manner, so as to preserve the health of the global environment. As such, we have lost the balance in our relationship to it.

Because humans have such a vast influence on the environment, the loss of the Keys of Health has led to erosion of the health of the natural ecosystems on our planet.

One of the bigger examples of this is the way we relate to the forests of the world. Our planet's well-being is greatly dependent on the forests that have a crucial purpose of creating oxygen, upon which all life depends. They are the lungs of the planet. They also provide a home for the vast variety of animal species on the planet. They support the soil by protecting it from erosion and sanitation. They themselves are a living element, which not only serves and aids animal life, but has a right to exist, because they form a healthy part of the ecosystem which creates life on Earth.

During the last few generations, humans have cut down forests at a rate that has never been seen in human history—much faster than they can be naturally regrown. We are destroying the forests of the world at around 1 percent per year. This rate of destruction has been going on since the 1970s and it's estimated that if this continues we will only have 10 percent of rainforest left by 2030, and none within a hundred years. This is not only extremely unhealthy, but a great tragedy that is largely going unnoticed.

> *In many ways, the human species is behaving like*
> *a pathogenic organism as it relates to the planet.*

We have structured our meaning around domination and self interest. We too often consider balance, if at all, only within the scope of human endeavor. We are slowly destroying the environment upon which we depend for our health, and are blind to our actions. We have to expand our vision and start creating in a healthy manner to stop this erosion of global health.

Yet because of the entanglement of health, we do not have to be superheroes and change the world. We simply have to understand what health is, begin to create health inside of us, and naturally it will ripple out into our environment.

Global Warming: Lack of Meaning, Balance, and Harmony

"I find it very sad that by the time corporate science realizes the value of nature, that it may be too late."

~ Steven Magee

Global warming is a symptom, a signal that the planet is unwell. Just like the human body develops a fever to signal it has an infection, so too the planet is signaling that health is being eroded. Unfortunately, scientific evidence is showing us that humans are the main cause of this illness.

Instead of seeking to contribute to the world and each other in ways that serve life, we have too often found meaning in the idea of "more". Simply thinking that having more is somehow what we are here for. Yet this ever-increasing growth is creating an imbalance in our relationship to the environment, and degrading the health of the natural world. This kind of action is throwing out the harmony, not only of nature, ecosystems, and animals, but the whole planet. It's echoed in what we know as Global Warming.

Yet unlike pathogens in a body—who are genetically programmed to act in an unhealthy manner—humans are unique. Our uniqueness lies in our ability to reflect on who we are, and how we are behaving.

We have a choice. We can choose again, to change, and recreate a new mythology. One that is congruent with health.

This is where this journey is taking us.

We have seen that the creation of health, and indeed the erosion of it, does not originate at the level of the cells, or the mind, or even on the well of global phenomenon. It is true that they influence each other in direct and indirect ways. But the causation lies deeper. It lies on the level of "Identity". It lies on the level of mythological understanding of who we are, and how we relate to the world. It resides inside a field of reality that is available to us, in all places, and at all times.

To truly understand health, we have to go deeper than our understanding of **what** it is, and **where** it is expressed. We have to understand its origins: **how** it is created and **how** we can reconnect to its flow.

So let us travel deeper now, below the surface of expression, and look at mythology. For in understanding our identity lies the key to how we, as individuals and as humanity, create ourselves.

In the next chapter, we shall see the ways humans have created an identity I call "Perceptional Reality", which lacks the keys that create health, and has led to the erosion of health in our expression, and the many sufferings we experience on the physical, social, and global scale. Once we understand the root of Perceptional Reality, we can journey towards understanding **how** the Keys of Health can be recreated in our own experience.

This process is embodied in the 12 Principles of Health that enable us to connect to the field of Vitality. They create the founding Mythological Identity that enables the expression of the Keys of Health in our life.

Vitality is a field of intelligence that animates matter using various energy sources to create a healthy living organism. As such, Vitality merges matter, intelligence, and energy—in a healthy manner. The 12 Principles of Health are the core intelligence or principles that are used in this process.

So let us journey deeper to discover the dynamics of *Mythology* that underpin our identity and creative potential.

Chapter Summary:

1) Disease manifests in the physical, social, and global spheres when the intelligence of health is lost in living organisms.

2) When meaning, balance, and harmony are eroded in cellular expression, then physical illness like infections, autoimmune diseases and cancer manifest.

3) When meaning, balance, and harmony are lost in our psychological expressions, social problems like racism, sexism, and war begin to manifest.

4) The loss of health in the body, mind and society affect each other in a direct fashion.

5) The causation of illness and health does not occur on the level of expression—it occurs on the level of identity. For health to manifest, our identity has to be congruent with its underlying principles.

6) Because humans have such a vast influence on the environment on a global scale, our inability to express ourselves in a healthy manner as a human species is slowly destroying the health of the world at large. This is seen in the destruction of natural ecosystems and global warming.

Chapter 3

Mythology: The Story of Who We Are

*"We shall not cease from exploration, and the end of
all our exploring will be to arrive where we started,
and to know the place for the first time."*

~ T.S. Eliot

On our journey so far, we have discovered that health is a meaningful, balanced, and harmonious relationship within, and between, living organisms. This manifestation is orchestrated on the level of the cell, the mind, and the environment in which we live . It is expressed in the body, society, and the world at large. Health is unified, animated and flows from a field I term "Vitality". We have seen that physical, social, and global illness manifest when the three Keys of Health are eroded, and unity is replaced by a conflicted divide.

This raises the questions:

— *How do living organism create the Keys of Health?*
— *How are they lost?*

To answer these questions we have to delve into the nature of individual living things, to look deeply at how they create themselves and their relationships. We have to explore the realm of mythological understandings, which hold sway underneath the surface of our conscious minds as they express the creative potential of living organisms. This place is where our identities are created. We have to go to the core of who we are, and from where we recreate ourselves.

Mythology refers to stories that define us. Who we are, how we relate to the world, and where we come from. They capture fundamental expressions regarding our beliefs, emotions, and relationships.

When we connect to Vitality and begin to understand the principles that life uses to create health, and express them in our own lives, we become empowered to start creating meaningful, balanced, and harmonious relationships in our own experience. It allows us to create a healthy relationship with ourselves, with others, and with everything else in our world. This understanding becomes the foundation of a healthy life—an embodiment of a healthy mythology.

Yet not all mythology is healthy. Because individuals have choice. We are empowered to see and interact with the world in any way we desire. When individuals are blinded to Vitality and do not understand the way health operates within them, they begin to make choices incongruent with the reality that governs health. This erodes our meaning, our ability to keep balance and create harmony, and expresses itself as illness. I term this mythological expression "Perceptional Reality". It is an absence of health flowing through matter.

Thus, let us look more closely at how our mythology is created.

Scripting Mythology: We Are the Creation of Our Past

*"We are products of our past, but we don't have to
be prisoners of it."*

~ Rick Warren

When you look at your life in a mythological manner, you begin to see your life as a story. We like stories because, in a very real sense, we are one. Yet in this magical tale that creates our life, there reside three key storytellers.

The first storyteller is our cells.

Cellular mythology is inherited through our genetics. The body has an innate intelligence passed on through our genetic code—a book holding nine billion pieces of information, called nucleotides. This code creates "words" called codons that are transcribed within the cells and translated into "chapters" called mRNA sequences, and then into physical matter. This process determines the physical components, and autonomic actions of the cells and the body they create. However, even though cells express health and disease in physical ways, it is the underlying intelligence governing these basic units of life that determines which expression takes place.

The second storyteller expresses itself through our psyche.

The psyche is the product of our minds. It is taught to us by our parents, teachers, relatives, and peers who script our beliefs and mold our perceptions as we grow up to become independent adults. It is here that we inherit the ideas of who we are, how we relate to each other, and the way we see the world as a whole. This story creates our personal and social understandings and molds our relationships. This scripting of our "identity"then influences our bodies because of the way we treat ourselves, and it also is expressed in the way we interact with others and society at large. In a very real way, psychological, social health, and disease is a product of the intelligence we express every day as a result of who we have been scripted to be.

The last story teller is created by the environment in which we live, work, and play.

Our environment is the co-creation of all living things. It creates the context through which we define ourselves on a day to day basis. If our environment is devoid of healthy expression, it affects our own health. If our environment is healthy, we are influenced in a healthy manner. As such, we are influenced by all of life that surrounds us, and the underlying mythological intelligence that created it.

It's interesting to note that much of who we have become has been created, or inherited, from our past experiences.

> *It is the narration of those who have come before us*
> *that creates our present.*

The foundations of our bodies is already scripted from genetic materials that have been passed on from our parents and their parents—a legacy passed down by our ancestors.

Our psyche is molded by our parents, teachers, and mentors that taught and influenced us as we grew to become adults. They, in turn, were molded by their parents, and so our minds are crafted from the heritage passed on by our ancestors.

The way we belong is crafted by the environment we grew up in, which was scripted and created by the collective consciousness of the society in which we live, and which has been created over many generations.

By the time we become adults, our beliefs, perceptions, and the values taught to us, create our thoughts, feelings, and behaviors. They shape the lens through which we see and interact with the world.

Our bodies behave in autonomous ways along genetic pathways that we have inherited. As such, to a large degree people become who they were molded to be. It is the choices made from our past—the choices of our ancestors who came before us—that script our mythological understandings and expressions that too often shape our destiny.

In an ideal world our mythology would serve us. Genetics would not be flawed and we would have inherited a healthy set of genes. We would have grown up in a supportive and healthy family, and been taught the principles of health. We would have matured to become independent adults capable of keeping balanced, and interacting in a harmonious manner. As a result, we would have learned to create healthy expressions and interdependent relationships with others, and with our world, that adhere to the Vitality that governs health. We would have created healthy environments, and would live and work in supportive systems that help us grow, passing on wisdom to the next generation.

Yet we live in a world that's not ideal.

> — *What if our paradigm drives us towards illness, to imbalance, and poor relationships?*
> — *What if our environments do not support healthy expressions?*
> — *What then?*

As humans we have been placed in a very privileged and unique situation. Because we are human, we have the capacity to transcend the choices and influences of our past.

Of all the living creatures on the planet, we possess the greatest ability to reflect on who we are, and what we have become, and then choose again to create our future—a new future.

Elephants possess the gift of strength, cheetahs are fast, and birds can fly. Humans are unique in their ability for **self-determination**.

Between stimulus and response we have made our stand. To choose who we are in relationship to the environment we find ourselves in. This unique gift enables us to take hold of our own destiny and create a healthy life in our own experience. We are the products of our past, but we need not be its prisoners. As humans, we have the power to recreate who we are.

Scripting Mythology: The Choice of Creation

"You are free to make whatever choice you want, but you are not free from the consequences of the choice."

~ Unknown

It is human awareness of one's self as an individualistic identity, relating to the world, which gives one the freedom to create any mythological construct one can imagine. This power enables us to **self-determine** our beliefs by reflecting on who we are in relationship to the world, and then "choosing" who we wish to be.

Our mind enables us to create our own mythology—not only to be a part of our environment, but to create it. Yet such power has become a double-edged sword. Without understanding the principles upon which health stands, it is easy to create mythological constructs that are deeply unhealthy. This has been an ongoing problem in human society.

For some reason, humans often disconnect from "Vitality" and the knowledge that governs the creation of health. Today, our influence as a human species on the planet is so great that we simply cannot continue to do this without dramatic and devastating consequences to life on the planet. We no longer just influence our own health by the choices we make, but the health of every other life form on the planet. Now, more than ever, humans need to reconnect. We have to reconnect to the essence of life from which Vitality flows.

Choice can lead us astray, yet choice enables us the freedom to change, and realign our lives with Vitality and the principles that underpin health. Choice is a gift requiring respect and understanding if it is to be used in a healthy manner that enriches life in a creative way, rather than resulting in a distortion of life's fundamental reality, leading to loss of health in all its expressions.

The good news is that the field of Vitality is already present all around us. It emanates from all living things.

Vitality cannot be corrupted, like the body, mind or environment can, because it is not changeable by the choices of our cellular, physical, or environmental realities.

Yet Vitality can influence all these aspects of ourselves to return back to a healthy state of expression.

— So why do we so often choose mythological constructs which are unhealthy?

To answer this question, we have to unlock the mythological construct that leads to illness. Before we explore the 12 Principles of Health that captures the intelligence of Vitality that life uses to create itself, we will look at the mythological constructs that erode health. Understanding this reality enables us to make choices to start to free ourselves from its influence and enable us to leave behind the scripting of **Perceptional Reality**. We can then embrace the flow of Vitality.

Chapter Summary:

1) Mythology describes our identity. It refers to stories that define us: who we are, how we relate to the world, and where we came from. They capture the fundamental beliefs, that lead to our thoughts, emotions, and the way we structure our relationships.

2) Our self Identity story is expressed on the level of the mind, the cells, and the environment.

3) Our "Identity" is inherited from our past. We are who we were scripted to be. Yet as humans we have a choice to recreate ourselves through the choices we make in the present.

4) Choice is a double-edged sword. We can create health by tuning into Vitality—the field that encodes health—or we can destroy it by creating via Perceptional Reality.

5) Understanding Perceptional Reality enables us to leave it behind and start our journey to understanding and creating health.

Chapter 4

Understanding the Mythology of Disease:
The Creation of Perceptional Reality

*"Perceptional Reality, is an expression of who we
are not"*

In our current Western medical health paradigm, disease is seen as an entity that is to be understood and remedied—or prevented—so that health can once again prevail. This has proven to be a useful and powerful approach that has alleviated much suffering in the world.

Yet the paradigm is incomplete:

> Health is seen as an *absence of disease.* However, when one looks closely at the reality of life, the exact opposite is true.

> When we look at "disease" through the paradigm of health, as described in this book, the mythology of disease in its essence is an *absence of health.*

In the mythological expression, the absence of health is created by a conflicted dualistic world I call "Perceptional Reality". When people get lost in Perceptional Reality they start to lose their internal meaning, lose balance, and express an unhealthy relationship with themselves, with others, and with the world as a whole. Harmony is eroded and replaced by conflict—they get lost in the shadow of their own Vitality.

Vitality is never affected by Perceptional Reality because it resides in a field of existence beyond the shores of individualistic perception. It is the "Keeper of the Flame" that forever holds the blueprint of health. When allowed to flow freely, Vitality creates a synthesis of mind and body that results in a vital, healthy, living organism. Flowing broadly, it can create a healthy world, yet it can be obscured when our minds and bodies lose sight of its wisdom and begin to script themselves with the mythology of Perceptional Reality.

Understanding Perceptional Reality

*"Perceptional reality does not see the world as it is.
It only sees its own perspective."*

~ David R. Hawkins

The Story of Socrates

It was mid-morning. Socrates had gone for a walk outside the city walls of Athens. He was at rest and about to eat his lunch, which he knew to be a masterpiece of Greek food, when a traveller hailed him.

"Greetings, friend!" he called. "Can you tell me, is this the right road for Athens?"

Socrates assured him that it was. "Carry on straight ahead," he said. "It's quite a big city, you can't miss it."

"Tell me," continued the traveller. "What are the people of Athens like?"

"Well," said Socrates, "Tell me where you come from and what the people there are like, and I'll tell you about the people of Athens."

"I am from Argos and I am proud and happy to tell you that the people of Argos are the friendliest, happiest, most generous people you could ever wish to meet."

"And I'm very happy to tell you, my friend," replied Socrates, "that the people in Athens are exactly the same!"

The traveller went on his way, and Socrates remained seated on his milestone. The conversation made him feel like celebrating the goodness and humanity in the world. He opened the wineskin resting at his foot to enjoy with the lunch he had prepared for himself.

Yet just as he was about to take a drink, another traveller came along the road.

"Greetings, friend!" called the traveller. "Can you tell me, is this the right road for Athens?"

Socrates assured him it was. "Carry on straight ahead," he said. "It's quite a big city, you can't miss it."

"Tell me," continued the traveller. "What are the people of Athens like?"

"Well," said Socrates, "Tell me where you come from and what the people there are like, and I'll tell you about the people of Athens."

"I am from Argos," replied the second traveller. "And I am sad and disappointed to tell you that the people of Argos are the meanest, most miserable, least friendly people you could ever wish to meet."

Socrates considered his response, then replied: "I am very disappointed to tell you, my friend, that the people of Athens are exactly the same."

~The Magic of Metaphor

Creating Perceptional Reality

When we begin to see life only from our own perspective, and begin to lose sight of Vitality and the innate experience that health is a unified reality—we create **Perceptional Reality** within our minds.

There are three fundamental beliefs that create Perceptional Reality:

1. *Perceptional Reality does not see our connection to life. It believes we are isolated.*

2. *Perceptional Reality sees meaning as external, and does not believe we have innate meaning.*

3. *Perceptional Reality believes life is polarized. That well-being is attained by winning.*

When we begin to see our lives in a perceptional way, we create a vacuum of meaning in our own experience, for we no longer see how we belong to life, and feel isolated. Because meaning is a fundamental key in life, we begin to seek meaning in the things outside of ourselves.

Things we label "meaningful" are considered "good", encoded as a feeling of pleasure, while things that keep us from these objects of desire are labeled "bad", and trigger a feeling of emotional pain.

Because meaning is perceived to be external, we need and desire that which we think will bring us meaning. In our materialistic society, this is often physical things or other people's affection. Yet, because we cannot fully control our environment or the actions of others, we script our reality in a dualistic manner: we **win** if we get that which we need and desire, and we **lose** if we do not.

The world is scripted in a similar manner, becoming polarized. The polarity creates conflict. We begin to believe that winning this conflict is the means by which we can attain our meaning and well-being. In reality the opposite is true. The polarity created by Perceptional Reality begins to erode our health.

First we lose balance.

The world appears as a binary reality of Good vs Bad. We support and cling to the "good" that we think will bring us what we need to fulfill meaning, and we fight the "bad", against anything that takes it away from us. Lost in the polarity of opposites, our experience sways from pleasure to pain, and we find ourselves unable to balance the psycho-emotional forces of life.

We become "victims" when the world does not give us what we think we need. We become full of pride when we "win" and lean towards intimidation and aggression to get—and keep on getting—what we desire. We lose sight of the natural balance of the seeming opposites that health depends upon.

This unbalanced experience erodes our relationships. Conflict replaces creativity and harmony. Instead of seeing the ways various elements come together to create a greater whole, we polarize them into conflicted divides. We are no longer creating our lives in a balanced manner from the innate meaning that springs from within. Instead we find ourselves in perceptional conflict with the world, grasping for external meaning that always seems to escape us. This destroys our ability to create in harmony.

Having lost internal meaning, balance, and harmony, we slip into an unhealthy reality. In our personal lives, we struggle to understand why we are here, feeling isolated. We find the world a place of conflict—often an angry place—a place that lacks meaning and cohesion. A world where struggle and conflict are the norm. This reality ripples outward, creating the social problems we experience in our lives.

This Perceptional Reality has sometimes been called the "flaw" in humanity. In the Buddhist tradition, it is called *Samsara*, meaning "illusion". In the Christian tradition it is has been called *sin*. The "illusion" is created by our ability to mis-perceive life.

Life, at its essence, is created through the power of healthy expression. It is a meaningful, balanced flow of harmonious relationships—a unified reality.

Perceptional mythology scripts the founding idea that life is based on conflict, and that health is found by winning this conflict. That we are separated from life, and need to "Win" the meaning we so desire. This reality places humanity in a matrix of perceptional creation, fighting to break free, and seldom realizing that it is the struggle creating the perceptions that obscures the flow of healthy expression.

How Perceptional Reality is Encoded in Psychological Reality

"We do not see the world as it is,
we see it as we are ..."

~ Anais Nin

The majority of Perceptional Reality is scripted below the level of our awareness—in our subconscious minds.

Perceptions, in essence, are beliefs with emotional significance that we hold to be true about ourselves, other people, and the world at large. These are incongruent with the reality of life, and thus health. These beliefs are held in the psyche by powerful representations of reality that are generalized and internalized. These are Representations, Generalizations, and Internalizations, or RIGs, and they color our personal experience of life, creating internal conflict that pulls us into psycho-emotional illness. This is reflected in our actions as external conflicts that create the social problems our society has found so difficult to deal with (see previous chapter for discussion on these social problems).

A simple example of a destructive RIG is: "*I am not worthy of other people's love*".

Running this belief will lead a person to subconsciously undermine their relationships. They may not even be aware they have this belief. It creates resentment and conflict and leads to a relationship breakdown. However, the belief itself is not real, for love is a fundamental element that creates life. Yet because one has adapted this distorted belief, the mind will try to create a reality from it. This is done by the way we think and feel, the way we treat ourselves, the way we treat others, and by choosing to relate to people who have complementary belief systems.

We often succeed in creating this reality, and the lie becomes the truth. As we live out our lies, our thoughts, feelings, and actions create a field of experience congruent with our perceptional error. It becomes held in our reality and influences all those around us. In a very real way, we become lost in a destructive matrix created by our subconscious minds that erodes our experience of health. The perception that we are not worthy becomes a perceived reality.

Matrix of Polarity: The Mythology of Duality

*"The superior takes credit for the good, the inferior
takes blame for the bad …
When they unite, love is created."*

~ Anais Nin

A Zen Buddhist Fable

Once upon a time there lived an old farmer who worked his crops for many years. One day his horse ran away. Upon hearing the news, his neighbors came to visit.

"Such bad luck", the neighbors said sympathetically.

"Maybe …" replied the farmer.

The next morning the horse returned, bringing with it three other wild horses.

"How wonderful!" The neighbors exclaimed.

"Maybe …" said the old man.

The following day, the farmer's son tried to ride one of the untamed horses. He was thrown and broke his leg. The neighbors again came to offer their sympathy on his misfortunes.

"Maybe …" said the farmer.

The next day, military officials came to the village to draft young men into the army. Seeing the farmer's son's leg was broken, they passed him by. The neighbors congratulated the farmer on how well things had turned out for him.

"Maybe …" replied the farmer.

Because balance is the nature of life, even in our perceptional realities we seek balance in our own experience. As such, if a person has a deeply negative perceptional view of the world, they create a positive fantasy that is the polar opposite of their belief.

For example, "I am not worthy of love", will be balanced by the fantasy of the "soul mate" that will give the "perfect love" they know is missing in their heart—this now becomes the meaning they seek. Their life experience may oscillate between these two polar extremes: thinking they found the "perfect one" only to realize that they too are just human, and then fall back into the disappointment of feeling "not enough" for such love. This is the perceptional roller coaster of duality. All the while, health resides in the center of this roller coaster, in the realization that love is a natural flow of expression we can bring to others.

At its extremes, Perceptional Reality drives people to become "vampiric" in their relationships. Through manipulation they seek to feed an insatiable thirst to gain the attention and resources of others to fuel their perceived needs and desires. This drives their perceptional meaning.

However, draining others of energy creates an imbalance in the relationship, and leads to conflict as the opposing polarity tries to rebalance the equation in an unhealthy manner. On the other side of the polarity we become as if a werewolf—openly attacking other's points of view, and fighting to impose our own worldview onto them. We may feel like "winners" for a while, yet we find life a hostile place as our "victims" fight back to regain what we have taken by force.

It's very difficult to see the flow of health when one is stuck in this polarized Perceptional Reality. Yet by its essence, the opposite polarity is a signal from life that we have lost our balance. It is a way to bring us back to the center for healthy expression to arise.

Perceptions are always created in pairs of imbalanced points of view. Like two sides of one coin they are forever linked, and forever in conflict with each other.

The stronger we **admire** creates the weaker we **avoid**.

The better we **strive for**, creates the worse we **fear of becoming**.

The higher we **reach**, the lower we **sink**.

The heaven we **cling to**, creates the hell we **fight against**.

There is no escaping the prison of duality within the walls of Perceptional Reality.
One can win some battles, but the war never ends.

The perceptional matrix is a prison that seems inescapable. This is because it is self-creating. The harder one struggles to escape it, the more trapped one becomes.

The only way out is transcending the whole paradigm, by stepping back and seeing the context of the situation, by choosing a "middle way".

Like in the Zen fable, the farmer understands the polarities of life, and knows that a healthy position is one that comes from the point of balance. At the center—the balance point—we find a doorway that opens to reveal our innate meaning that drives our purpose, and enables us to become creative in the way we relate to the world. The result is an increasing harmony that unifies us to the world we live in. In a very real way, we begin to transmute unhealthy experiences into healthy ones.

Exploring Perceptional Reality: Social Constructs

*"All the world's a stage, and all the men and
women, merely players ..."*

~ William Shakespeare

The main problem with Perceptional Reality, is that it creates an underlying subconscious mythology that creates a whole paradigm of experience, making it difficult to see the "center" from which the flow of Vitality can be experienced.

Stephan Karpman, a prominent psychologist and one of many thinkers who observed the way Perceptional Reality is created within the experience of social interaction, called one such experience the "Drama Triangle". This construct describes the way we experience Perceptional Reality in our conscious awareness.

The drama triangle is created by a Victim, a Persecutor, and a Rescuer. Because perceptions are founded on the polarity of good and evil, one side becomes deemed a victim, and another a persecutor. The persecutor is perceived as the villain and the victim as an innocent. The rescuer plays the hero, who tries to bring victory to the side that is deemed "good". Yet because the paradigm is fictional—or perceptional in its essence—each player has a covert motive that is actually benefitting egoically in some way. As such, they don't seek solutions or a way to create in a healthy manner because their meaning is sourced from the drama. Once this perceptional template is set, endless stories can be created from its perceptional paradigm, yet the ending is always the same. Some battles are won, but war never ends.

When we explore the key error, we begin to see that the archetypal drama triangle is created when meaning is sourced from perceptional duality, or from an external source.

The Persecutor is egoically rewarded for being stronger that the victim, for the ability to manipulate and control them, which is perceptionally desirable and meaningful. They have become a "winner".

The Victim is rewarded because they have the moral high ground and thus feel entitled to the support or rescue of others. Their meaning is one of righteousness.

The Rescuer is rewarded because they are scripted as the savior of the innocent, and is therefore elevated in their position.

Yet, as Transpersonal Analyst Claude Steiner noted: "The victim is not really as helpless as he feels, the Rescuer is not really helping, and the Persecutor does not really have a valid complaint."

The whole perceptional game is fictional and can be very destructive to our health.

The reason this mythological construct is unhealthy is because the relationship of victim, rescuer, and persecutor is one of codependency. They depend on each other to source perceptional meaning from their given positions. The rescuer keeps the victim dependent on them by playing into their victimhood. The victim gets their needs met by having the rescuer take care of them. The persecutor is required to keep the game going, and is rewarded for strength and getting their way.

In this codependence of meaning, real solutions are overlooked. To have their emotional needs met, the disfunction of the perceptional game must continue. Balance and harmony are forsaken for conflict and perceptional meaning. Unless meaning is found elsewhere, the players are trapped in the dysfunctional game that is not congruent with psycho-emotional health. Indeed, it is the source of conflict.

When one is deeply scripted in Perceptional Reality, the payoff from playing these games acts like an emotional magnet that keeps us locked into this way of seeing. It's only when we discover a deeper reality, with a higher meaning value, that we look back and smile at the childish nature of such destructive games. It's not until we can see through the "illusion" of perceptional conflict—into the world of principles that describe the way health is expressed in living things—that we begin to escape the matrix we have created.

The Experience of Perceptional Reality

"Your perspective on life comes from the cage you were held captive in."

~ Shannon L. Alder.

We have discussed the subconscious and conscious mechanisms that create Perceptional Reality—yet how do we experience them?

Our experience of Perceptional Reality is often simply emotional in nature. This emotional experience then drives our thoughts, and unhealthy actions. The whole paradigm is held together by strong emotional bonds that represent the underlying construct of beliefs and ideas about who we are and how we belong in the world.

On the extreme side of victimhood, we experience apathy and depression, the feelings of worthlessness and lost hope. We live with *anxiety* and *fear* as we see the meaning we desire but cannot grasp it. We continuously find ourselves on the losing side of the conflicts we experience. We are driven to escapism through addictions to substances like alcohol and other drugs to keep our anxieties at bay—if only for a while—yet drive us deeper into illness. We wallow in a sense of helplessness.

These strong emotions reinforce the perceptional matrix and drive our thoughts and actions—or inactions—that keep us in an unhealthy way of being. We blame the "evil" in the world for our problems, and hope that a savior may one day come to free us from the perceptional prison we find ourselves in.

On the other side of the Perceptional Reality coin, we experience emotions of anger, rage, and hate as we seek to take by force that which we think we need to secure the meaning of our desires. When we find ourselves "winning", we experience pride and judgement of others. We feel like we are better, stronger, and more deserving than others. We cling to this false sense of confidence as it gives us the emotional feeling of winning the battle. Yet this polarization always leads to conflict, and often our downfall. Those we try and suppress rise up in rebellion, aided by the saviors who come to their rescue.

Even the savior is caught up in a sense of pride for representing the "good" side, and battling "evil" in the world. Yet their meaning is sourced from this pride, and so evil has to exist for their meaning to be fulfilled. In a subconscious way, they too hold the unhealthy experience in place.

Because there is an interconnection of life, perceptional polarities always create their opposites to balance the experience being created.

Perceptional Reality creates a paradigm of intelligence that creates the loss of health. On the psychological level it creates destructive relationships. At its extreme it manifests as sexism, racism, and even war. When Perceptional Reality is expressed in the intelligence of our bodies, physical disease is made manifest. When it ripples out into the world it creates the great global challenges facing us today. The source of all this is made manifest, not from a causation, but from the identity of life.

Letting Go

"Sometimes letting things go is an act of far greater power
than defending or hanging on."

~ Eckhart Tolle

We have reached a basic understanding of Perceptional Reality, created on the founding belief that life is a polar experience of good and bad, and meaning is found in the stuff of life. It is a reality that:

- *is reinforced by subconscious beliefs that support this model, held in place by strong emotional bonds that reinforce the "illusion" that Perceptional Reality will lead us to win back our health*
- *masks internal meaning, destroys our balance, and prevents us from creating harmony in our relationships*
- *makes us believe we are separate from life, and that life is founded on conflict between individuals, where spoils go to the victor*
- *erodes health on the physical, psychological, social, and environmental levels, as the unity of life falls to pieces that find themselves in conflict with each other.*

The question then arises:

- *Now that we understand the reality that keeps us from health, how can we step out of Perceptional Reality and step into the flow of Vitality to create health in our experience?*

It's time to let go, and it will be okay.

A Two-Step Process

There are two steps to this process—two steps to change the way we experience and create our lives—that can set us on a path to creating health in our own experience.

The first step is to understand and let go of that which does not serve us anymore. To understand and let go of Perceptional Reality, which creates unhealthy expressions in our body and mind.

The second step is to understand and embrace the principles of health that encode the expression of Vitality in living things. To step into the flow of Vitality, which creates health in our bodies and minds.

Letting Perceptional Reality go is best done on an emotional level, for it is our emotions that lie closest to the subconscious scripting of our bodies and minds. They encode a vast array of thoughts, words, and stories that play out the perceptional matrix in our experience.

However, the understanding in our minds is not enough. One has to translate psychological understanding into a visceral experience.

To fully step out of it takes our ability to feel the emotions that hold it in our reality and let them go.
To simply say: "No".

People react in three ways to perceptional emotions:

1. They express them, which reinforces their reality, such as reacting with anger that drives conflict.

2. They suppress them into their subconscious, which drains their energy and leads to apathy and depression.

3. They seek to escape them through substances of addiction, which numbs—if only for a while—the

experience of the pain that results from the conflict being created.

The path to letting go is simply to observe our perceptional emotional expressions with the knowledge that they are not who we really are. They are not congruent with health, with life, or with the essence of our vital self. We observe them without judgement. We do not express them, suppress them, or try to escape them. We simply observe them to understand what lies at the heart of their expression.

When we do this, just like clouds on a summer's day, they begin to dissolve and disappear over time because they were never our true reality in the first place. They are not congruent with the nature of life, or healthy existence, that lies at the heart of living things.

This process of letting go creates space within us. Through this space, we start to get a glimmer of the flow of Vitality, which emanates from life, from ourselves. It is at this point we become ready to begin step two. The adaptation of health principles, upon which health is founded.

Chapter Summary:

1) When an individual loses "sight" of Vitality, they begin to see the world from their position only. This creates a mythological construct called "Perceptional Reality" that erodes health in the individual's experience.

2) "Perceptional Reality" does not see the world as it is—it only sees its own perception.

3) "Perceptional Reality" does not see our connection to life, and believes meaning is external.

4) The loss of inner meaning drives polarized and unbalanced action, which creates conflict that erodes harmonious relationships.

5) In our subconscious experience we perceive expression of Perceptional Reality as victim-mentality, aloofness, intimidation, or aggression. This is reflected in our subconscious as vampiric, or werewolf tendencies.

6) In the social dynamic, the drama triangle is an example of a construct based on Perceptional Reality. The interplay between victim, persecutor, and rescuer drives and defines our meaning, eroding healthy social relationships.

7) To create health, one has to let go of Perceptional Reality.

Chapter 5

Stepping Into Our Health Creation

"A healthy outside starts from the inside."

~ Robert Urich

When one studies life—and thus health—closely, we begin to see that it is not founded on perception. It is founded on key principles. These principles transcend conflict and lead a person on a journey towards something mysterious. It is mysterious because life is in constant movement, growth, and flux. It cannot be captured in a perceptional manner. It's almost like one starts to step into a moving stream of life that flows in a harmonious way. Yet this river flows from inside of ourselves and spills out into the world.

The journey starts with the realization that life is not perceptional. It evolves as we let the perceptional world go and begin to find one's own **independence** or inner meaning and balance. It proceeds on through to **interdependence**, or the ability to transform differences into synergistic, mutually-beneficial relationships, that are balanced, harmonious, and which unify life. Moving deeper, one begins to sense the "Sanctum" of one's soul—a reality from which life and health flows. It is here where the answers to health reside.

The journey is not a journey of becoming "better, bigger, or stronger". Those are the victories of the perceptional paradigms, which by their very definition lead to "poorer and smaller", as it is visible in the human social construct.

It is about expanding one's vision of life—from a black-and-white perceptional paradigm founded on the battle between good and evil, to a colorful dimension founded on principles that enable creative synergy, through to a place where words end and experience begins. The spectrum of health bends through the prism of our being, coming into a unity from which Vitality flows into our experience.

Vitality resides at the intersection of physical matter, intelligence, and energy. It brings these three elements together to **animate** health.

So, let's embark on this journey now by exploring the paradigm shift required to reach this place where health becomes a natural state of being.

Health Paradigm Shift

"The way we see the problem is the problem."

~ Stephen R. Covey

Three Stonemasons

During the early years of the fourteenth century, the foundations of a magnificent cathedral were being laid in central Europe. The Clerk of Works was a monk charged with the task of supervising all the laborers and artisans. The monk decided to carry out a study into the working practices of the stonemasons. He singled out three stonemasons whom he thought were representative of different attitudes towards their profession.

He approached the first stonemason and said:

"My brother, tell me about your work."

The stonemason stopped for a moment and replied in a clipped voice, full of anger and resentment:

"As you see, I sit here in front of my block of stone. It measures a meter, by half a meter, by half a meter. And with every blow of my chisel against the block I feel as if I am chipping away a part of my life. Look, my hands are callused and hard. My face is lined and my hair is grey. This work is never ending, the same, day in, day out. It wears me out.

Where's the satisfaction? I'll be long dead before this cathedral is even a quarter finished."

The monk approached the second stonemason:

"Brother, tell me about your work."

"Brother," replied the stonemason in a soft, even voice, "as you see, I sit here in front of my block of stone. It measures a meter, by half a meter, by half a meter. And with every stroke of my chisel against the block I sense I am carving out a life and a future. Look, how I am able to shelter my family in a comfortable house, far better than that in which I grew up. My children attend school. No doubt they will look forward to even more in life than I do.

All that is made possible by my work. As I give to the cathedral through my skill, the cathedral gives to me."

The monk approached the third stonemason:

"Brother" he said, "tell me about your work."

"Brother," replied the stonemason, smiling and in a voice full of joy, "as you see, I sit here in front of my block of stone. It measures a meter, by half a meter, by half a meter. And with every caress of my chisel against the block I know that I am shaping my destiny. Look, see how the beauty trapped within the form of this stone begins to emerge.

Sitting here, I am celebrating not only my craft and the skills of my profession, but I am contributing to everything that I value and believe in, a universe—represented by the cathedral—where each gives of his best for the benefit of all.

Here, at my block, I am at peace with who I am, and I am grateful that, although I will never see the completion of this great cathedral, it will stand a thousand years, a beacon celebrating what is truly worthy in all of us, and a testament to the purpose for which the Almighty has put me on this earth".

The monk went away and reflected upon what he had heard. He slept more peacefully that night than he had ever done, and the next day he resigned his commission as Clerk of Works and apprenticed himself to the third stonemason.

~ The Magic of Metaphor

This story is a metaphor that captures the three key paradigms people embrace when they look at health and disease in their experience. Sometimes the way one *sees* a problem, *is* the problem. So too, is it with creating a healthy life.

First Paradigm: Survival of the Strongest

The first, and least useful paradigm, is founded on the idea that life is a battle—the strongest survive. Because of this perception, health is seen as the ability to destroy disease. If a person adapts this way of seeing health, illness becomes an enemy to be fought. As a consequence, life becomes a struggle, and health is seen as a victory. A world of winners and losers is created, where only the strong survive. A never ending battle of good and evil.

These ideas, founded on the paradigm, shape our experience. We begin to feel this way. Our ideology about health and disease becomes this way. We struggle to kill cancer, to destroy microorganisms, to defeat incurable disease.

This model can be seductive in its simplicity and blinding in its intensity. Yet when one takes a step back and looks at it from a distance, it has a deep, fundamental flaw—a blind spot which actually hinders a person from being able to lead a healthy life. The flaw is that it does not see the reality of health. It does not understand that **illness is conflict**. It is founded deeply in Perceptional Reality. Trying to fix conflict with conflict cannot work in reality.

Disease can be defeated in some instances, battles can be won, but the war never ends. The paradigm does not have the power to create a truly healthy lifestyle.

Albert Einstein once wrote that a problem can't be solved at the same level as it was created. So too it is with creating a healthy life: one cannot solve it from within the paradigm of conflict, for disease is a conflicted relationship.

Therefore, a new paradigm must arise. As Stephen R. Covey a best selling author once wisely commented: "Sometime the way we see the problem, is the problem."

Indeed, the way we see the problem must change.

Second Paradigm: Science and Allopathic Medicine

The next level of mythology regarding healthcare is captured through the scientific paradigm. We stopped seeing disease as an enemy that needed vanquishing, and asked ourselves the question:

— *What is this thing called illness anyway?*

The **mythology of understanding** was the dawning of science. Science is a paradigm of thinking founded not on the idea of a battle of Good vs Evil, but one of understanding of life. The enemy is "ignorance".

Understanding disease processes allows us to intervene in creative ways to restore biochemical functioning and structural integrity, correcting disease expression in the process. It's the platform on which allopathic medicine was founded. Its power comes from the paradigm itself, because once you understand a problem you can act on the process in a fashion that works to fix it. Yet the paradigm is focused on the distortion of illness, and therefore is limited in its ability to provide health as a desired end point. As a result we have mountains of knowledge on thousands of disease processes.

We have hundreds of ways of "fixing" problems that we now understand in their mechanism. Yet illness is just as prevalent now—if not more so—than it was in the past, even though our ability to manage illness has seen exponential growth. Major diseases like type 2 diabetes, heart disease and depression have seen ever increasing growth in recent decades. And as health budgets reach breaking point, people start to ask the question:

— *What is the way forward?*

Once again, a new solution has to arise. A solution founded on a different way of seeing the problem. The solution is the creation of a new paradigm that humanity is looking to embrace. This paradigm has the capacity to evolve healthcare because of the intrinsic power it holds. It is the understanding of health itself.

Third Paradigm: Health Creation

The third paradigm is the understanding of health itself.

— *What if the solution to illness is not destroying illness, or not even understanding and fixing illness?*
— *What if the solution to creating a healthy life, is choosing health?*
— *What if health could be understood, and its essence could be embraced?*

When one breaks down the elements of health, it becomes apparent what health actually is. We have seen health is not a battle. It's not even a form of understanding—it's a love story. Health is a harmonious relationship of balanced independent elements that serve each other for the greater good of life. Its foundation is the meaning that lies at the heart of life.

When one embraces this paradigm, one can start to ask oneself:

How is love created?

The movement to love is the movement to health. That's where the focus has to be. Yet love is not only a feeling, it's a way of life, a way of relating.

So what is this thing called love anyway?

Could it be that we as humans are seeking not to have more, not even to understand more? Maybe we are seeking the peace that flows through a loving relationship. We are seeking health, because we know it is our nature. We are the health that we are looking for.

Having studied medical science and medicine for more than a dozen years, one begins to see something about the nature of health:

Health is real. Health is not a perception. It's a principle.

Let us take our journey further into a deeper dimension of understanding. Let us leave the world of conflicted Perceptional Reality as we walk away from the pendulum of duality. Let us journey, under the surface of the psycho-emotional ocean of Perceptional Reality, to discover a whole new world—a new mythology—on which health is founded.

As we journey, I hope you notice that it is not the world that changes, it is ourselves. Yet as we change, the world changes with us. And as we arrive back at the beginning—back to who we are deep down—we cut through the haze of our perceptional identity and begin to become aware. We return to the place we started, and know it as if for the first time.

Chapter Summary:

1. Changing from creating our lives in a perceptional manner, to creating our lives in a healthy manner requires a paradigm shift.

2. The "Survival of the strongest" paradigm sees the world as a place of conflict, in which health can be found by destroying the evil in the world. It is deeply perceptional.

3. The paradigm of science, seeks to understand and solve the problems of the world, so that a healthy expression can result. It is a useful and powerful paradigm, but limited because its focus is on problem solving, rather than the creation of health.

4. The "Health Creation" paradigm seeks to understand the underlying "Intelligence of Health" so that it can be created in our experience.

Chapter 6

The 12 Principles of Health: Exploring the Intelligence of Health

"I'm trying to free your mind, Neo. But I can only show you the door. You're the one that has to walk through it."

~ Morpheus in the movie The Matrix

The Lighthouse Story

Once upon a time, a powerful battleship was patrolling a strategically important coastline at night. In the distance a light was spotted by the ship's scouts. The captain was notified and he immediately got onto the radio to contact the other vessel.

"This is an order to the vessel directly in front of us," he said with a voice that resonated with authority. "Divert your course fifteen degrees South to avoid a collision."

After a short pause a reply came: "We recommend you divert your course fifteen degrees North to avoid a collision".

The captain was startled. "Don't they know who we are?" he snapped angrily at the other vessel's disrespect.

He gave a quick reply: "This is the Captain of a battleship. We have right of way. You must divert your course fifteen degrees South to avoid a collision!"

There was a short silence before a calm voice replied over the radio: "Negative, Captain. You will have to divert your course fifteen degrees North to avoid a collision."

The Captain's patience ran out.

"This is the Captain of the most powerful battleship in these waters. We have a fleet of ten warships in our wake. I insist you divert your course fifteen degrees South or you will be fired upon and destroyed!!"

After a brief pause, the reply came in as calm a voice as before.

"This is a lighthouse. It's your call."

~ Unknown source

Principles are not perceptions—they are real, fundamental aspects of life. They are the intelligence that govern the physical, psycho-emotional, and energetic elements upon which healthy life is founded. They are like lighthouses signaling the path home, standing on the foundation of life itself.

Where **perception** can be stronger, bigger, better, and bend a person's mind to their way of seeing, **principles** have the power to restore health to our lives. They do this by making us aware of who we are deep down below the surface of our Perceptional Reality.

The story of the battleship and the lighthouse is a metaphor that illustrates the difference between perceptions and principles. Perceptions are like ships that roam the waters of the psycho-emotional landscape. Some are very powerful and influential. The lighthouse, however, is like a principle that represents a certain reality of life. Its position is stable. It is aligned with reality. It does not fight because it understands that health cannot be found in conflict. Yet it cannot be fought either, for nothing that is real can be destroyed. It can only be acknowledged, and as such, can lead one to safer waters.

Principles are not enemies of perceptions. Yet without them, perceptions often end up shipwrecked on the rocky shores of life.

PRINCIPLE 1
You Are the Creator of Your Reality:
AWARENESS

*"Your thoughts are not who you are.
You are the awareness that has power to control
what you think."*

~ Unknown

Invictus

*Out of the night that covers me, black as the
pit from pole to pole,*

*I thank whatever gods may be, for my
unconquerable soul.*

*In the fell clutch of circumstance, I have not
winced nor cried aloud.*

*Under the bludgeonings of chance, my head
is bloody, but unbowed.*

*Beyond this place of wrath and tears, looms
but the horror of the shade,*

*And yet the menace of the years, finds, and
shall find me, unafraid.*

*It matters not how strait the gate, how
charged with punishments the scroll.*

*I am the master of my fate: I am the captain
of my soul.*

~ William Ernest Henley

Experiencing Awareness

My first vivid experience of **Awareness** came in the midst of great misfortune.

In a real sense, my world was falling apart. I lost my job, the relationships I cared for were broken or breaking, and my ill health was slowly eroding my dream of a meaningful life. I experienced so much emotional pain and blamed the world for the way life was treating me. I was so lost in the conflict that I could not see where I was anymore. I felt I had tried everything, but I simply could not win ...

I sat on a beach consumed in sorrow when something unique occurred to me.

I am not sure why, but perhaps it was because I had tried all the combinations of a lock that simply would not open, and I finally surrendered to my predicament. I allowed myself to see the pain I felt inside without judgement or feeling the need to fix it.

I stopped fighting. I stopped projecting the cause of my pain onto others. I simply followed it into myself and observed what was at the core of its existence. Sometimes grace manifests, and that day was such a time.

Suddenly the pain and grief started to disappear and I found myself in the eye of my emotional storm. I saw all the turmoil in my life around me, yet my consciousness was no longer affected by it. I found myself in a calm and peaceful place. There was great meaning there. It was the first time I truly experienced the realm of Vitality vividly. As it moved in my mind, I could see the illusion of my own Perceptional Reality that was running my life.

I saw that the storm that had caused so much pain in my life was not real. I had found **awareness** of a reality outside of Perceptional Reality.

From this place I knew I could move my psycho-emotional world in a meaningful and constructive manner. A great joy came over me—a joy that had no relationship to the mess my life was in. It was meaning flowing from within.

I suddenly felt I could stay balanced, as I was no longer being blown over by the powerful emotional waves created by my subconscious mind. Instinctively, I knew that from this place I could be the master of my own fate, I could be the captain of my destiny. I did not know how, but I knew it was the first step to recreating my life.

The Principle of Awareness

The first principle of health is founded on an innate reality that resides within all living things—a reality that creates health within living organisms. I call this realm of experience **Vitality**.

The principle of Awareness denotes our ability to "tune in" to this invisible, yet very real aspect of our own being. It is through Awareness of this place that we realize there is an internal guidance system available to us that is always seeking a healthy reality in our experience. We also become aware that we have the ability to choose the way we see and react to the world around us. We begin to see that we are not our thoughts, beliefs, or perceptions. We are not the thoughts, beliefs, or perceptions of others. Instead, we are the Awareness observing these thoughts and beliefs, and choosing which ones will govern our expression and determine who we become. In this Awareness resides an innate intelligence that understands how health is created, and leads us to express this in our own lives.

Awareness is present in all living systems.

Because life only exists by the grace of its ability to create healthy pathways, Awareness is available in all places, and in all moments of our lives. It arises from life itself—in the silence of the moment—and seeps into our consciousness.

Between stimulus and response, humans can make a stand: Instead of reacting in perceptional ways, looking for a cause of blame, we have the ability to pause and reflect, and become aware that we can choose who we are in relationship with the world of circumstance with which we find ourselves. We can stop reacting and start creating ourselves in a healthy manner. It is here, at the creative edge of our life that awareness can open up a door to our health creation.

When we start our journey to find a healthy life, often much is beyond our control. Unless we have been lucky and have grown up in a healthy family environment, we find obstacles that we need to overcome. Genetics influence us, subconscious psycho-emotional programs we have unconsciously learned run us automatically, and the environment we live in forces us to react in conflicted ways at times. Our reactions are often unhealthy, and we experience this as conflict and pain.

Yet as we begin to understand and feel the nature of health, and realize we have the power to choose our own destiny, we start to have a glimmer of hope—or a foot in the door, so to speak. We have a realization that we do have the key to shift from someone who reacts to the world, to a person who is creative in the way they relate to their life. From someone stuck in a Perceptional Reality that does not serve them, to someone who can choose balance, unearth their innate meaning, and take a journey deeper to unlock the secrets of creating harmony in life.

From the vantage point of awareness, we can create internal space to change who we are, how we relate, and what we stand for. We are empowered to stop reacting and consider the most fundamental questions:

— *What am I thinking?*
— *What do I believe?*
— *What do I feel?*
— *How shall I act?*
— *How can I align myself to create a healthy life?*

Awareness is revealed when we suspend our perceptional habitual reactions to our life. We begin to observe reality from a deeper vantage point and start to make conscious decisions about who we will become in relationship to all the thoughts, ideas, and actions we are experiencing from others, and from without our own minds and bodies. As we stay in this place, we sense the flow of Vitality that guides us to align our lives with healthy principles.

People who have founded their lives on this principle of Awareness stop blaming circumstances, conditions, or conditioning for their behavior. They start taking responsibility.

They do not blame the world or the storms kicked up by time and circumstance. Instead, they seek to create the weather of their psycho-emotional world and carry it with them. They understand the old wisdom:

It is better to light a candle, than to curse the darkness.

Indeed, they receive insight into that darkness we fear. They know it is not as real as imagined.

When a person begins to sense the flow of Vitality they no longer seek "more" as a way to define their worth, because they know that who they are holds far greater value and meaning than what they have, and so they journey to become more real. They become responsible and able to respond to the world in a constructive and healthy way.

Awareness is the first principle because it is the foundation upon which the whole construct of a healthy mythology stands. Without it, we are unable to connect to the source of health inside of us. Without it, life becomes confusing, conflicted, or our fate appears to be simply a matter of chance that rarely smiles upon us. A whimsical comedy of the Gods, perhaps.

Having found the "eye of the storm", we discover the peace and stillness from which guidance is available. It enables us to start making choices different from those we made in our past. We begin to change and undertake a journey towards creating a healthy life.

We can now build a whole new foundation on which our mythological reality can stand. We begin our journey to becoming masters of our own destiny, and creators of health in our own experience.

PRINCIPLE 2
The Strong Boundary:
SECURITY

*"You will not break loose until you realize that you,
yourself, forge the chains that bind you."*

~ Gary Renard

The Man, the Boy, and the Donkey

A father and his son were on the way to market with their donkey. They walked alongside the donkey, chatting about what they would buy that morning. As they were walking along the road to town, a countryman passed them by and with a tone of indignation he said: "You fools, what is a donkey for but to ride upon?"

The father stopped and considered this remark. He put the boy on the donkey, and they went on their way.

But as soon as they were approaching town they passed a group of men, one of whom shook his head and jeered: "See that lazy youngster? He lets his father walk while he rides! What is our youth coming to these days?"

The father stopped and considered this remark. He ordered his boy to get off, and got on himself. Satisfied, they continued on. But they hadn't gone far when they passed two women milling at the gates of the town. One looked up and said to the other in a loud voice so all around could hear: "Shame on that lazy lout to let his poor little son trudge along while he rides like a king!"

Well, the man didn't know what to do. He got off the donkey and looked at his son, who just shrugged his shoulders.

After a while he got an idea. He got back on the donkey and lifted his boy up before him on the donkey. Together they rode into town on their way to the markets. Yet they had not even reached the center of town, before a crowd of students started calling names in their direction. The man stopped the donkey and asked the student what they were scoffing at?

One student said: "Aren't you ashamed of yourself for overloading the poor donkey of yours— you and your hulking son?"

The man and the boy got off and tried to think of what to do.

They thought and they thought, until at last they cut down a pole, tied the donkey's feet to it, and raised the pole and the donkey to their shoulders. They went along amid the laughter of all whom they met.

The father finally realized the absurdity of the situation. He untied the donkey and gave it a pat on the nose.

He looked at his son and said: "Whatever we do, someone disagrees with it. Perhaps it's time we made up our own minds about what we believe is right."

~Joseph Jacobs, The Fables of Esop

Experiencing a Strong Boundary

When I was younger, life puzzled me. Everyone seemed to have an idea of what was in my best interest, and for the world in general. The problem was that the ideas kept contradicting themselves and created conflict and confusion—that was until I understood Perceptional Reality and how easy it is to see life only from one's own perspective.

As my awareness grew, and I realized the power to create a healthy life lay within me, I asked myself:

> — *Who am I in relationship to all of the events that are occurring in my life?*

I started to create my experience of life, rather than try and find a perceptional answer that so often ended up in conflict.

The answer to this question crystallized with my experience of Vitality. The meaning, balance, and harmony that flowed from that place of Vitality I experienced on that beach that fateful day, was so rich and powerful I decided to mold my life upon the qualities that were present within it. I began a journey to understand the nature of what I had experienced. It was at the start of this journey that it dawned on me that in order to achieve this, I would have to say "No" to all the perceptions that were incongruent with this state of being—even if it meant changing my entire character.

I required a **strong boundary** that would allow me to create myself from within.

As I built this boundary, I stopped becoming as reactive to life events as I used to be. Life was not throwing me about like a feather in the wind, in all sorts of directions. My gaze shifted from a conflicted past and desirable future, to a creative and rich present. I became more responsible for my life. I was listening to the world and learning from it, and how I responded was my own choice and my responsibility, which governed my experience of life. I did not have to buy into its judgements, or define myself by my past failings. I was finding that this **security** gave me more independence and the ability to build myself into the kind of person I had always known I was capable of being. It enabled me to grow from the inside. I started to walk in the direction of my own destiny guided by my awareness. My journey had begun.

The Importance of a Strong Boundary

Living in a perceptional world can be hurtful and confusing. By trying to please everyone we often end up pleasing no one and become more confused. Similarly, when we try to do whatever we like without consideration for others, we create so much conflict that we are unable to do anything useful. This is why having a strong psycho-emotional boundary is so important.

A strong psycho-emotional boundary is created by the realization that who we are is not fundamentally determined by the perceptions of others or our own perceptions. Rather it flows from a deeper intelligence that encodes the reality of how living organisms create themselves in a healthy manner. Moment to moment, when we see that perceptional thoughts and ideas are not the real descriptors of who we are, they lose their ability to control us. We can say "no" to their influence. When this happens, we find our security, for we become free to change ourselves from the inside—to make new choices about who we are and how we will live life.

Security is founded on the first principle of Awareness because it is Awareness that helps us realize that who we truly are lies deeper than our thoughts. As such, our thoughts become our servants, not our masters.

A strong boundary frees us from having to buy into the perceptions of the world. It gives us permission to redefine who we are in relation to the world and others in any given moment. We start to see clearly that we hold the key to the chains that keep us locked to an unhealthy reality. From within the security of a firm boundary, we become free to choose to base our lives on the principles that support life, rather than the confusing and often contradictory perceptional realities of others—and indeed our own.

Once we have a strong boundary we become free to consider situations from a broader perspective, and to create new visions for our own lives. We become free to listen and seek to understand the opinions and ideas of others—those who may see or know things we do not— without feeling threatened by their thoughts. We can consider these opinions, information, and ideas, and choose to accept or reject them based on their merit, and in accord to the manner they relate to our lives.

> *Life is a unified concept after all, and wisdom can*
> *be found in all of its expressions.*

Saying "No" to Perceptional Reality

The **Security** of a strong psycho-emotional boundary enables us to say no to perceptions that cannot capture the truth of how to create our lives in a healthy manner. Just like in the story of the man and the donkey, there is no "real" true perception—all perceptions are always relative to the circumstances of one's life.

A famous Taoist saying illustrates this concept:

> *"Right and wrong are situational.*
>
> *In the appropriate situation, nothing is wrong.*
>
> *Without the appropriate situation, nothing is right.*
>
> *What is right in one case is not what is right in another.*
>
> *What is wrong in one case is not what is wrong in another."*

This statement illustrates that Perceptional Reality, which operates in the dualistic world of right and wrong, cannot capture the reality of life, and thus, health.

Life is more complex than this. It is fluid, and changes with circumstances. Yet its foundations never change. These principles that support health in any given moment cannot but capture health, for they are its reflection. Life is health and perceptions have to adhere to principles if they are to be life-supporting.

A strong psycho-emotional boundary creates a sense of simplicity and control in our lives. One's mind is no longer carried away on the roller coaster of perceptional duality. It becomes increasingly centered and focused—or **balanced**—in its outlook. It allows us to live more gracefully in an ever-changing world of perception and circumstance.

> *A strong psycho-emotional boundary requires us to*
> *suspend our judgement.*
> *There is no need to judge that which is not real.*

What we judge we often keep in our reality. Instead, what is required is to simply leave it behind and choose to create a new reality. In this process we learn that our worth, our happiness, and our sense of peace will not depend on the perceptions of others. Circumstances and opinions change. Indeed, our perceptions and opinions will also change. Yet our worth and our meaning are innately part of who we are. Like Awareness, it flows from within.

From this secure position we can create the foundation of our independence and inner balance. It is the **security** we require to have the integrity needed to build interdependent relationships that create the harmony upon which health is founded.

PRINCIPLE 3
Emotional Equanimity:
INNER POWER

*"If you change the way you look at things, the
things you look at change …"*

~ Dr. Wayne Dyer

The Guest House

This being human is a guest house.

Every morning a new arrival.

A joy, a depression, a meanness.

Some momentary awareness comes

As an unexpected visitor.

Welcome and entertain them all!

Even if they're a crowd of sorrows

Who violently sweep your house

Empty of its furniture, still, treat each guest
    honorably.

He may be cleaning you out for some new delight.

The dark thought, the shame, the malice.

Meet them at the door laughing

And invite them in.

Be grateful for whoever comes.

Because each has been sent as a guide from beyond.

By Rumi

Finding My Inner Power

I had found my security. I was building my life and growing along the pathway of who I knew I was capable of becoming. Yet for some strange reason, it seemed like the world wanted to get in my way. Someone would tell me what they thought I should do, and I would simply keep my council, and they would respond with anger and attack my point of view. I felt myself reacting emotionally, defending myself. Suddenly I was in an argument about what I believed and what they believed. Conflict seemed unavoidable. I could close my boundary, but somehow this made people more upset. It felt isolating. I felt myself sliding emotionally back into anger and frustration. I knew I was missing something.

Suddenly, as I was hiking through the picturesque landscape of Sydney's Blue Mountains pondering this dilemma, a story I read many years ago came to mind:

> A Buddha is sitting under a tree when a man approaches and starts to verbally abuse him, saying that the Buddha's teaching are all lies.
>
> The man continued for some time becoming increasingly angry and frustrated, but the Buddha did not reply.
>
> Finally the Buddha said to him: "If a man gives you a gift and you do not accept it, what happens to the gift?"
>
> The man was confused by the Buddha's question, but answered: "It goes back to the man who gave it."
>
> "Yes," said the Buddha. "So you came here and brought me anger and judgement. Thank you, but I do not accept them."

Suddenly the answer became very clear to me. There is no need to react emotionally in a conflicted manner.

There are things I am obliged to do within the bounds of society and it is indeed healthy to contribute to life, and stay balanced within its physical parameters, but no one can tell me who to be.

Life is like a dance and I began to notice that as I danced, so too do the drums beat. So I let the music of life be. There was no need to take it personally, fight against it, or cling to it. Instead, allow it to be as it is, and focus on my "dancing".

As my ability to do this increased, I found a new sense of balance in my life. Not only psychological balance from developing a strong boundary, but an emotional balance from growing in my own "power".

A **power** was born from my ability to keep **equanimity** in the way I viewed situations. A balanced emotional position that enabled me to see situations clearly and respond to them in creative ways that were constructive and fruitful, rather than react in conflicted ways that only brought havoc to all I had worked so hard to build.

As I changed, I observed the magic of the world changing with me—I began to notice the creative and mysterious nature of Vitality.

What Is Healthy Power?

The perception of power created by our egoic perceptional mind is power over others, not power from within. The Ego has a need to control that which is beyond its boundary to control, seeking dominion over others. The result is experiencing emotional pain and conflict when this control is not granted, leading to frustration, or grief, as one "burns" one's emotions by focusing on what one cannot control. In Eastern tradition, this is called suffering.

This path can lead to aggression as we impose our will upon others to give us what we desire. However, aggression often leads to retaliation and the end point is conflict, and relationships that are incongruent with health. This can also lead to a sense that we have lost our meaning, as that which we desire is not granted.

Where the ego sees "power", in reality there stands the circumstances that pull us towards psycho-emotional illness.

Healthy power is born from our Awareness to observe our Ego—the creator of Perceptional Reality. As we observe its movements within, we can make a conscious decision not to buy into its illusionary view of the world. Instead, we can choose to seek power over ourselves, not others.

Power over ourselves constitutes the ability to maintain **Equanimity**. Equanimity is the ability not to internally fight against what we don't like, nor to grasp for that which we do. When equanimity is attained, we simply accept what comes, and observe and learn from its presence. We realize that "resistance against" or "clinging onto" are us trying to do the impossible.

It is impossible because healthy living things are free in their essence, and trying to fight this freedom is incongruent with health. As a result, a person gains the ability to not take life personally. **This becomes a form of inner power—the ability to choose how to respond to life in a constructive manner.**

When we choose equanimity, we have the clarity to stop asking: *What is right?* or *What can we can control out there?* and instead begin asking:

— *What is healthy?*
— *Who am I to become in relationship to what is?*

As we start to eliminate emotional conflict in ourselves, we start to consider not what can make us win, but what can maintain our health. For our health includes their health too, and health is our greatest asset.

This ability to maintain equanimity is a process that takes place in the present moment. It is a way of "seeing" events in our lives, not as good or bad, but as things needing to be understood so we can relate to them in a healthy manner. As in the saying by the twentieth Century American author and poet, William Arthur Ward:

> *A pessimist complains about the wind,*
> *An optimist expects it to change.*
> *A realist adjusts the sails.*

It is our ability to see events with equanimity that allows us to adjust ourselves to it in a healthy manner. Inner power is another foundation principle that helps us construct our independence.

Where the Security of the second principle of strong boundaries creates **psychological independence**, the Power of the third principle creates **emotional independence**. Below the scripting of Perceptional Reality, humans are driven by principles. Meaning, this kind of power is natural, although it may not be normal as yet.

Equanimity allows a person to look at a greatly undesirable perception and consider it with **balance** and calm contemplation, and seek to find a resolution to meet the needs and desires of one's self and of others. It allows us to resolve the undesirable perception in a meaningful and harmonious manner. One begins to create the quality of composure to handle conflict in a healthy way, creating stability in one's emotional core. This gives us freedom to stay flexible to change and be creative in the way we relate to life. As life *is* change, this becomes a key principle of healthy growth.

In The Guest House story, Rumi likens ourselves to a guest house; one that welcomes in all new arrivals—be they of a joyful or sorrowful nature, and suggests we meet them all "honorably". Such acceptance enables us to understand the current paradigm we find ourselves in and recognize our guests are simply reflections of this reality.

This understanding enables us to let go of perceptions that do not serve us anymore.

The power of equanimity allows us to accept our current reality, creates the space required to let go of that which does not serve us, and grow toward the principles that create health in our own experience.

PRINCIPLE 4
Self Governance:
Balancing the Hemispheres

"The rational mind is a faithful servant: the intuitive mind a sacred gift. The paradox of modern life is that we have begun to worship the servant and defile the Divine."

~ Albert Einstein

On Reason and Passion

Your soul is oftentimes a battlefield, upon which your reason and your judgment wage war against your passion and your appetite. Would that I could be the peacemaker in your soul, that I might turn the discord and the rivalry of your elements into oneness and melody. But how shall I, unless you yourselves be also the peacemakers, nay, the lovers of all your elements?

Your reason and your passion are the rudder and the sails of your seafaring soul. If either your sails or your rudder be broken, you can but toss and drift, or else be held at a standstill in mid-seas. For reason, ruling alone, is a force confining; and passion, unattended, is a flame that burns to its own destruction. Therefore let your soul exalt your reason to the height of passion, that it may sing;

And let it direct your passion with reason, that your passion may live through its own daily resurrection, and like the phoenix rise above its own ashes.

I would have you consider your judgment and your appetite even as you would two loved guests in your house. Surely you would not honor one guest above the other; for he who is more mindful of one loses the love and the faith of both.

Among the hills, when you sit in the cool shade of the white poplars, sharing the peace and serenity of distant fields and meadows—then let your heart say in silence, "God rests in reason". And when the storm comes, and the mighty wind shakes the forest, and thunder and lightning proclaim the majesty of the sky—then let your heart say in awe, "God moves in passion". And since you are a breath in God's sphere, and a leaf in God's forest, you too should rest in reason and move in passion.

~ By Khalil Gibran

Finding My Psychological Balance

When I started to apply the first three principles of health in my life, I discovered a new sense of calm. It was a kind of inner space that was seldom there before. I realized I had spent a lot of time in conflicts with myself and others, chasing dreams, and running from things I did not desire. Suddenly, with these principles, I had an inner space to set a vision for my life—a kind of metaphysical potential you could say.

But what would I do with all this new space?

When we ask a question of the world and have the patience to wait, the answers often seem to present themselves out of nowhere, as if through chance or serendipity. The answer to this question was that this space is an opportunity to create something. Since health is a process of creation, I realized this act of creation was founded on another principle of health.

The human mind has two hemispheres, each with very different ways of operation. There is the hemisphere of reason or logic, and there is the hemisphere of emotional creativity. Until that time, my life was a tug of war between these two forces: my reason pulled me on one path, and my creative, passionate mind pulled me in an opposite direction. Yet now I could see that what I "perceived" to be conflict within myself was meant to be **cooperation**.

I had to balance my hemispheres and become a creative person in the way I approached my life. I could use my creativity to envision new pathways in my life, and use my reason to create a structure around this vision that would frame it within the context of my life. In so doing, I began to eliminate conflict between these two powerful forces, and unite them to drive my creative potential.

Balancing Creativity and Reason

The fourth principle of health denotes a person's ability to become a leader of their own lives. When we become aware of our ability to tune into a healthy reality, and find our own security and power, we can use these to begin to create our lives in a healthy manner. We start this process by balancing the hemispheres in our own minds.

When we examine the function of the cortex part of the brain, which is responsible for higher thought in humans, we can see two distinct parts of the mind: the left part of the brain thinks in terms of reason and logic. It looks at a problem and seeks to find a solution. Its function is characterized by sequence, order, and linear thought. It can put parts together into an organized whole. Its thinking is the essence of academic success as it is presently measured.

The right part of the cortex thinks in the spectrum of creativity and intuition. Its function is holistic and diffuse. The left brain instinctively sees the whole first, then the parts which create it. The right brain is founded in nonlinear thinking, such as dreams. As such, it is highly creative. It is capable of harmonious artistic expression.

Where the left hemisphere is linear, the right is nonlinear. The left is logical, the right is creative. The left operates in the realm of analysis, the right in the realm of creativity. The right solves problems logically, the left sees the problem holistically. The left uses math to explain structure, while the right is perceptive, intuitive, and sees what lies beneath. The left expresses itself through writing and reading, the right through dancing, music, and poetry. The left uses facts to attain goals, the right uses feeling to attain art.

The left values systematic order, the right values intuitive symbology. The left creates budgets and policies to govern, while the right uses wit and creativity to deal with each situation. The left uses objective planning to guide one's action, the right uses fantasy and spontaneous action. The left is traditionally masculine in its energetic essence, and the right is feminine, and only together, when the two hemispheres function in a balanced and integrated manner, does wholesome human function occur, and psycho-emotional health prevail.

When we look at the function of the two hemispheres we begin to notice why it is so crucial for their integration: the left brain is much like a computer, which strives to do things right. As such, it leads best in doing things, organizing things, planning things. It can create laws that serve any given system. Whereas the right side of the brain specializes in doing the right things. It sees the whole, understands the best way to relate, and as such, what actions are required in any given circumstance, for health to prevail.

When these seeming opposites come into balance they co-create in a healthy manner.

The right brain envisions the greater vision that serves the whole in a harmonious manner. The left brain then creates systems around that vision, which can be created in a linear manner in the physical reality. Together, they serve to create a healthy world.

When we contemplate the world through our right, creative minds, we take on a leadership role in our own lives. We feel the bonds of relationships and the flow of life. We can explore the balance of relationships through our creativity and imagination. This lays the foundation towards **synergy**, which we will discuss in further chapters.

Having realized the healthy thing to do, we can execute the decision though our left brains, which simply focus on doing it right, by organizing our actions in time and space in an orderly fashion. The left brain enacts the decisions of the right brain through its systemic functioning and organization skills of physical matter. This relationship ensures that health does the right things in the right way. As such, **balancing** the cortical hemispheres of our own mind creates the psychological harmony required to create a healthy life.

Balancing our hemispheres also allows evolution to happen in a healthy manner.

The right brain keeps us connected to the unlimited creative potential of relationships, seeking to expand, grow, and evolve. The left brain keeps us connected to the practical limitations of the physical world: what we can do, what we can afford, what best way to manage our time, ensuring we don't lose balance as we grow.

Because healthy life is growth within the confines of stability, this balance is an integral part of health. When our cortical hemispheres are balanced and operating in synergy, humans can experience the ability to be creative and expansive, yet grounded and productive.

Khalil Gibran likens the mind to a ship sailing on the ocean of life. The left brain is like the rudder that keeps the ship stable and on course. The right brain is the sails of the ship that catch the winds of passion and circumstance to sail towards our destiny. Only together can life progress passionately and effectively. Without a sail we are stuck in the doldrums of reason, and without a rudder we tend to lose control and often end up shipwrecked in a storm of misguided passion.

Looking more broadly, science is founded on the technical left brain and art is founded in the creative right brain. They both have to meet in a synergistic fashion to create something more than the sum of their parts, and to capture the nature of health.

When we observe any healthy life form, we can see this synergy in action. Imagine a tiger hunting in a forest—looking with the eyes of reason we admire its anatomy, habitat, and evolutionary adaptation as a hunter. Looking with the eyes of creativity we feel its raw power, frightful beauty, and passionate intensity. Together, they capture the reality of a healthy tiger.

*Imagination was not meant to be used to escape
life, but to create it.
Reason was not meant to create life, but to organize
it.*

PRINCIPLE 5
Emotional Alchemy:
Creating Happiness from Within

*"But what is happiness except the simple harmony
between a man and the life he leads."*

~ Albert Camus

The Parable of the Lost Son

"There was a man who had two sons. The younger
son said to his father: "Father, give me my share of
the estate." So the father divided his property
between them. Not long after that, the younger son
got together all he had, set off for a distant country
and squandered there his wealth in wild living.

After he had spent everything, there was a
severe famine in that country, and he began to be
in need. So he went and hired himself out to a
citizen of that country, who sent him to his fields
to feed pigs. He longed to fill his stomach with the
pods that the pigs were eating, but no one gave
him anything.

When he came to his senses, he thought: How
many of my father's hired servants have food to
spare, and here I am starving to death! I will set
out and go back to my father and say to him:
'Father, I have sinned against heaven and against
you. I am no longer worthy to be called your son;
make me like one of your hired servants'. So he got
up and went to his father.

The son said to him: "Father, I have sinned against heaven and against you. I am no longer worthy to be called your son; make me like one of your hired servants". He then got up and went to his father, but the father said to his servants: "Quick, bring the best robe and put it on him. Put a ring on his finger and sandals on his feet. Bring the fattest calf and kill it. Let's have a feast and celebrate, for this son of mine was lost and is found again." So they began to celebrate.

Meanwhile, the older son was in the field. When he came near the house he heard music and dancing. He called one of the servants and asked him what was going on. "Your brother has come home," he replied, "and your father is holding a celebration because he is back safe and sound."

The older brother got angry and refused to go in. His father went out and asked him why he was so upset. "Look, all these years I've been slaving for you and never disobeyed your orders. Yet you never even gave me a young goat so I could celebrate with my friends. But when this son of yours who has squandered your property with prostitutes comes home, you kill the fattened calf for him!"

"My son," the father said, "you are always with me, and everything I have is yours. But we should celebrate and be glad because this brother of yours was dead and is alive again; He was lost and is found."

Luke 15: 11-32

Finding My Happiness from Within.

At times in my journey I felt alone. When one changes, one's relationships also change, and this can bring loneliness, a sense of anxiety, and fear.

For every door that closes, another opens, but the corridors in between can seem long and lonely places. Perhaps that is why many people stay in lifestyles that are unhealthy, rather than risk change.

Taking a surf on one of my favorite beaches I thought to myself:

> — *Who would risk the comfort of the known—even if it no longer serves you—for the unknown? How can one solve this dilemma?*

I stared at the waves rolling into the beach, tuning into the Vitality that I was able to access more and more often. Suddenly, I realized the answer was right in front of me: The waves were being created by the ocean as a natural flow of life. Perhaps happiness is created from within, and also has a natural flow.

I had always assumed that happiness came from what you had, or at least from the relationships you had. Surely happiness was a function that came from the world ... but suddenly I wasn't so sure anymore.

Vitality is innate in all living things. It animates from life. Since I was alive it must be flowing from within me also.

Could I find a sense of well-being, regardless of my life's circumstances? Could I harness courage, regardless of what success or failure life may be presenting me. Could I flow well-being and courage into the world and create my happiness from within?

Suddenly the matrix of my mind inverted:

> — *What if happiness is something I could bring to a healthy relationship, instead of being something I sought to gain from it?*
> — *Would this not take me a step closer to emotional freedom, to a healthy and meaningful life?*

This moment was the dawning of my emotional independence. It made logical sense.

— Yet how could it be achieved?

As always, life inevitably presents the answer.

What Is Happiness? Where Does It Come From?

In the world of perception, happiness is derived from getting what we want. We perceive that satisfying our desires will make us happy. Because perception is dualistic in its structure it often becomes a pursuit of having "more"—or at least more than the person next door. It is often about being "better", or at least "better than" our perceived opponent.

Perceptions also seek to control others, and so happiness is often tied to how others act towards us.

Is this real happiness or is it the never ending pursuit of having more, being better, stronger and controlling others? Perhaps a mirage in the desert of perception?

In the story of the lost son, one son pursues happiness by spending his wealth, yet ends up broke and miserable. The other son stays true to his duty and position, yet pursues happiness in seeing himself better than his "lost" brother, and loses his perception of happiness when his brother is exalted. The father, however, understands that happiness comes from an internal source. He is happy to give and celebrate with both sons, even when they perceptionally seem to betray or grow angry with him.

The mythology of the lost son points to a place of happiness that derives from within. So let us explore this happiness the father has.

Shifting to Emotional Alchemy

In the realm of principles, happiness is the emotional experience of living a healthy life. It is an intrinsic quality of living organisms. It is our nature; it springs from our Vitality. Therefore, happiness is created as the layers of Perceptional Reality are removed from our experience. I call this shift in attention: **Emotional Alchemy**. It is the transmutation of negative, painful, unbalanced emotions into a balanced outlook with a natural joy within.

Emotional alchemy can be seen as balancing the cortex of the brain with our limbic system—the part of the midbrain where emotions are generated.

In the fourth principle we balanced the hemispheres of the cortex, harmonizing both the creative and logical aspects of the mind to become creative leaders in our own life story. Now we triangulate, and harmonize with our limbic system, so that it balances with our higher cortical thinking.

In many people, the limbic system—the generation of our emotions—is perceptionally scripted, it generates positive and negative emotions based on desirable or undesirable external circumstances. Yet at its core, it has the capacity to create a sense of happiness as a natural outlook regardless of the circumstances of life.

The first step to this natural creation of happiness—to practicing emotional alchemy—is to adapt the first four principles of health. This creates space within us, allows us to say no to perceptional thoughts and emotions, and to take a leadership role in creating our life. When we achieve this, we can become creative in the way we create our emotional experience of life.

— *So, how does this occur?*

Two of the most common perceptional emotions that humans experience are **anxiety** and **anger**. The process of emotional alchemy can be used to transmute these two powerful emotions back into a sense of happiness.

Persistent anxiety arises when one has a deep psycho-emotional grounding in Perceptional Reality—the ever-changing life can provoke high anxiety. "What is right?"

"What is wrong?" is constantly changing. The fear of judgment and failure also increases anxiety.

However, persistent anxiety becomes highly dysfunctional to life. It stops us from taking action and from being creative, making a bad situation even worse.

Anxiety is also "contagious". As such, life becomes a mirror, where the anxiety we feel is adapted by those around us and projected back onto us. To make matters worse, our brains encode neural pathways that are memories of how we respond to life. When anxiety becomes learned it becomes a habit and takes on a biochemical imprint, which makes it much more difficult to undo, because it simply becomes the normal way we perceive the world.

Perceptional Reactions to Anxiety

When anxiety is experienced, people react in three primary ways depending on their psycho-emotional programing. This programming may be influenced by genetics, by what we learned growing up, and by our environment.

The first perceptional reaction is one of suppression. We suppress the anxiety. This is created by a great desire to escape the discomfort. Yet suppression of anxiety into our subconscious mind ignores the problem, and therefore, the feeling continues, and resurfaces in various life circumstances that we attract into our life because of the underlying wound.

The second perceptional reaction is to try to escape anxiety. This is done through addiction to substances that suppress the internal discomfort of anxiety. Alcohol, drugs, medications, and people, are just some common forms of addiction. Yet the addiction creates a downward spiral, as the anxiety only increases each time the substance of addiction wears off. It only elevates the disfunction and creates more anxiety.

The third perceptional reaction is to project anxiety into our world. To avoid the pain of looking at the source of the anxiety, we instead project it outward and blame the world for the way we feel. Yet this blame game is an emotional maze, as if made of mirrors with no way out. The more we see anxious events in the world around us and blame them for our anxiety, the more anxious we become.

Because we can't change the world, the cycle of anxiety only escalates in intensity, and we feel helpless to rid ourselves of its dysfunctional effects. People often shift from suppression to addiction to blame, as they fight to escape anxiety through perceptional pathways.

The Path Out of Anxiety

The path out of this perceptional prison of anxiety is to face reality as it stands—to become *aware* that we have the ability to find a solution. An internal solution.

It takes a great deal of **security** and **power** to do this. It also takes the ability to **self govern** to create solutions to the problems we face. This core stability created by the first four principles allows us to face what it is that makes us anxious, and decide who we will become in relationship to it.

Taking the action to deal with the source of our anxiety is **courage**—the courage to accept that which we cannot change, and instead focus on taking healthy action in our lives. To act in accord with the principles of life, and kickstart the journey back to innate meaning, inner balance, and a healthy creative life.

The actions made from this kind of courage make us realize we have the capacity to **change**, to become proactive and creative, and to meet the challenges of life. As we ground ourselves in the **awareness**, **security**, **power**, and **cortical balance** from within, we find the **courage** to act, and anxiety transmutes to **confidence**. Confidence that we can manage our own lives in a healthy manner. Thus, **confidence** becomes a key ingredient in finding happiness in one's own experience.

We can now move forward with a new resilience and begin to rewrite the scripting of our own minds, and re-create our lives, and ourselves.

Perceptional Reaction to Emotional Pain

On the other side of the spectrum of emotional imbalance is **hurt**, or emotional pain, that reflects as the emotion of **anger**. When people become hurt by the world they respond in three ways.

One way is to suppress the hurt.

This suppression is a kind of resignation of the perceptional attack bestowed upon us by others or ourselves. The suppression is done to avoid looking directly at the source of the hurt. However, it leads to a spiral of negative perceptions that dampen emotions resulting in feelings of apathy and depression.

Depression can arise from other places, including physical illness and biochemical imbalance in the mind, yet from the psycho-emotional aspect of the spectrum it is created from suppressing hurt, which creates the deflated feeling of depression. The depression then makes us see the world through a filter of negativity, which drives the hurt to be revisited on us in a spiral fashion. Escaping this "gravitational" pull of negativity becomes increasingly difficult as the mind sets up neural patterns, that replay a **victim-perpetrator relationship**.

When **hurt** becomes conscious, many people do not accept the hurt they feel because it is a very uncomfortable sensation. The fear of facing it leads them to project the hurt onto the world and other people. This projection leads to anger, blame, and even conflict, as this psycho-emotional reflex only leads to others fighting back.

The perceptional mind creates an internal Good vs Evil story and thus defends its position. This creates a cycle of conflict and ongoing hurt. However, the fight has no winners. It is a closed loop of hurt, fear, anger and conflict. Some world conflicts have been stuck within this doomed cycle of destruction for decades—if not centuries.

The famous quote from Yoda in the *Star Wars* series captures this phenomenon:

> *"Fear is the path to the Dark Side.*
> *Fear leads to anger, anger leads to hate, hate leads*
> *to suffering."*

Fear is the fear of not facing one's hurt, and suffering is the result of living in a conflicted relationship with the world and with one's self.

When we practice **emotional alchemy** we stop suppressing hurt. We stop projecting it into the world. and seek to transmute it into well-being.

Path Out of Emotional Hurt

To create well-being from within, a solid, independent, psycho-emotional foundation has to first be laid. By embracing **Awareness**, internal **security**, **power**, and **cortical balance**, as described in previous chapters, we set the stage for emotional transmutation of anger. This process is one of **affirmation**—affirming who we are in principle. We realize that no one can tell us who to be, but that we can create our own well-being.

When we look directly at who we are—without the perceptional filter—we begin to see the reality of our situation. We are, in fact, the health that we have been seeking.

Our bodies are created from thirty-seven trillion cells, living their reality in an interdependent manner, where innate meaning, balance, and harmony prevail the vast majority of time. All that is needed is for us to affirm our reality.

We are not the negative polarised perception bestowed upon us by the misguided minds of others, or even by our own mind. We are human living beings, whose lives are literally founded on love and creativity.

By affirming who we are, we transmute **hurt** into **well-being**.

The well-being that flows from this shift of focus is another foundation in our ability to create happiness from within: together, **well-being** and **confidence** create the emotional state of **happiness**. Joy is the natural awareness of who we are. It's already within us. We are the magic on which this alchemy is founded.

In his book, *Seven Habits of Highly Effective People*, Stephen Covey wrote:

> "But remember: if we search deeply enough within ourselves, beyond the scripting, beyond the learned attitudes and behaviors—the real validation of happiness and every core principle is in our own lives."

This quote captures the essence of **emotional alchemy**.

> *Health is who we are, and joy is simply the experience of this reality.*

Having balanced our cortex with our limbic system, we have gained another principle towards creating our independence and taken another step towards our health creation. Now we start to ask the question:

— How do we belong in this life?

This question is the driving force of individual meaning and leads to the final principle upon which our **Independence** is founded.

PRINCIPLE 6
Finding our Uniqueness:
Guidance

"To be born is to be chosen. No one is here by accident. Each of us was sent here for a special destiny. When you can awaken this sense of destiny, you come into rhythm with your life."

~ John O'Donohue

The Animal School

Once upon a time, the animals decided they must do something heroic to meet the problems of the "new world", so they organized a school.

They adopted an activity curriculum consisting of running, climbing, swimming, and flying.

To make it easier to administer the curriculum, all the animals took all the subjects.

The duck was excellent in swimming, in fact better than the instructor, but he made only passing grades in flying, and was very poor in running. Since he was slow in running, he had to stay after school and also drop swimming in order to practice running. This was kept up until his webbed feet were badly worn and he was only average in swimming. But average was acceptable in school, so nobody worried about that except the duck.

The rabbit started at the top of the class in running, but had a nervous breakdown because of so much make-up work in swimming.

The squirrel was excellent in climbing until he developed frustration in the flying class where his teacher made him start from the ground up instead of from the treetop down. He also developed a "charlie horse" from overexertion and then got a C in climbing and a D in running.

The eagle was a problem child and was disciplined severely. In the climbing class he beat all the others to the top of the tree, but insisted on using his own way to get there.

At the end of the year, an abnormal eel that could swim exceedingly well, and also run, climb and fly a little, had the highest average and was Valedictorian.

The prairie dogs stayed out of school and fought the tax levy because the administration would not add digging and burrowing to the curriculum. They apprenticed their children to a badger and later joined a groundhog and gophers to start a successful private school.

~ George H. Reavis

Who am I? What do I stand for?

These questions were always at the back of my mind. I was always one of those "all-rounder" persons, throwing my hat into many an endeavor. At school I played in the concert band, played chess, and soccer. I liked science, but also enjoyed geography and history, and joined in all the annual school musicals. I wanted to know and learn it all. Yet there was always an unanswered question growing louder in my subconscious mind as the years rolled on. It whispered: "Who are you? What do you stand for?"

As I matured, the answer slowly began to take shape. I was someone who enjoyed solving problems, who enjoyed being creative, and helping people. Someone who wanted to understand everything I could.

After completing my science degree at the University of Sydney, I realized science was too dry for me, too analytical. I applied to do medicine, which seemed more congruent with who I was. Yet it took many years to realize that my passion was not really in solving the problem of disease, but in understanding the mystery of health.

There came a time in my life several years ago, when I had an epiphany—a moment of profound clarity. I suddenly realized my uniqueness was my keen interest in understanding the mystery of life and what lay at the heart of its creation. I wanted to understand and share what health was! Not just physical health of the body, but the vibrant health of the mind, and the greater health of the planet as a whole.

This realization turned my paradigm upside-down. For so long I had been trying to understand disease and how to fix it, and now I realised it was Health Creation that I was seeking. I had found my uniqueness and it emanated from within.

From this place arose a well of unseen meaning that propelled me forward. The path has been rocky and twisted, and at times slow, yet inside there was a bright amber glowing—a fire that would never go out. Its meaning fuelled my purpose.

Without knowing my uniqueness I was too often driven by seeking pleasure, avoiding pain ... now I was free to embrace pleasure and pain in equal measure, driven to fulfill a deeper purpose that echoed from within. It became the outward expression of the independence I was finding inside myself.

This is another principle of health.

Exploring Our Uniqueness

On this journey towards health creation we have taken responsibility for our own experience of life. We have created **security** by creating a **strong boundary** and gained **inner power** by learning to observe the ego, and not to take **Perceptional Reality** personally.

We have **balanced the hemispheres of our cortex**, so as to engage our left brain in aligning our actions with what is congruent with health, and our right brain in organizing our lives in a practical manner. Through this we have gained the ability of **self governance**.

These principles establish an independent core within us, and allow us to engage in **emotional alchemy** so as to integrate our limbic system and create happiness from within. This has placed us in a position to move outwards and choose a life of meaning that is congruent with who we are. This principle is founded on the innate uniqueness of all human beings.

We all have strengths, weaknesses, and characteristics that shape us in different ways. We are inspired by different things. We think and create in unique ways. Some of us are inspired by art and creative endeavors, others by reason, logic, and structure. Others by bodily kinesthetic endeavors, such as sports. We find ourselves pulled by different passions in different fields of life.

> *The field that suits us will move us. It will make us feel inspired. It will feel not like work, but like a challenging game.*

We are able to become good at what we do because we love it.

Creating a life that is congruent with one's uniqueness is fundamental. This is because the innate **meaning** that drives our **uniqueness** is a core principle on which psycho-emotional health is founded.

There is no doubt of the importance of being grounded in the foundational aspects of psycho-emotional reality, such as reading, writing, scientific, and mathematical thinking. These are founded in reason. Artistic expression is founded in creativity and the wisdom of our own spiritual nature. These are present in all cultures.

It is also prudent to be worldly, to understand the historical and political positions, and environmental situations of our world. Yet each of us are drawn to a given area of expertise—an area of passion and interest that sparks our imagination and inspires our reason. Finding one's **place** within the structure of our society is a key principle of health. This **place** denotes the roles we play in the game of life. It's what we give to the world.

Our uniqueness, like our happiness, flows from within us. It becomes the expression of our innate meaning, which we can bring to the world. It is the sixth and last principle that forms the creation of our own **Independence**.

— *Where does this uniqueness exist?*

The great mythologist Joseph Campbell captures the essence to this answer in his quote:

> "Life has no meaning. Each of us has
> meaning and we bring it to life.
> It is a waste to be asking the question when
> you are the answer."

A Worldwide Health

Because life is a unified reality, our uniqueness naturally harmonizes with the broader ecosystems and social paradigms to which we belong. It makes us active players in the great game of life. Yet, we are also evolving.

As we grow, as our awareness expands, and our relationship to the world deepens, our uniqueness also evolves. The pinnacle of such growth is our ability to not only be great at what we do, and find our place within the human social structure, but to *create* it, in an ever more meaningful and healthy way. This ability to create our social structure is what enables us to change old, outdated models of thinking, and to embrace new ways of seeing that are more congruent with reality.

Humanity is moving towards an ever-increasing ability to create whatever we have the ability to imagine, yet it must be done in a way that is healthy—that is, aligned with the natural world and the principles of health.

In the field of healthcare, I believe the path should focus on creating a healthy society. As we leave the world of perceptions and build our social structures on the principles of health, we are creating a society founded on health: *A Worldwide Health.*

Our uniqueness is found as we journey towards creating a healthy life. Our uniqueness will find us, for it is a founding principle upon which health stands. It is always whispering in our subconscious, waiting for us to tune in and listen.

This spirit of our own uniqueness is captured by one of the great personalities of our age, Buckminster Fuller. With these words he captured the essence of this health principle:

> *"Never forget that you are one of a kind. Never forget that if there weren't any need for you, you wouldn't be here in the first place. And never forget, no matter how overwhelming life's challenges and problems seem to be, that one person can make a difference in the world. In fact, it is always because of one person that all changes that matter in the world come about. So, be that one person."*

SUMMARY OF PRINCIPLES 1-6

Creating Independence

*"Because you have a high degree of security,
guidance, wisdom, and power
that flows from a stable unchanging core, you have
the foundation of a
highly proactive and highly effective life. "*

~ Stephen R. Covey

We have reached half way in our exploration of the principles of health.

The combination of these first six principles create an independent core within us. This is the foundation of healthy relationships. They can be seen as the **masculine half** of the health paradigm—the place where strength, power, internal happiness, balanced thought, and a sense of mission in life arises.

Before moving on to the next six principles—the world of interdependent relationships that create the **feminine half** of the principles of health—we can pause and reflect on the foundational character created by the embodiment of these six health principles captured in this famous and timeless poem:

IF ...

IF you can keep your head when all about you

Are losing theirs and blaming it on you,

If you can trust yourself when all men doubt you,

But make allowance for their doubting too;

If you can wait and not be tired by waiting,

Or being lied about, don't deal in lies,

Or being hated, don't give way to hating,

And yet don't look too good, nor talk too wise:

If you can dream—and not make dreams your
    master;

If you can think—and not make thoughts your aim;

If you can meet with Triumph and Disaster

And treat those two impostors just the same;

If you can bear to hear the truth you've spoken

Twisted by knaves to make a trap for fools,

Or watch the things you gave your life to, broken,

And stoop and build 'em up with worn-out tools:

If you can make one heap of all your winnings

And risk it on one turn of pitch-and-toss,

And lose, and start again at your beginnings

And never breathe a word about your loss;

If you can force your heart and nerve and sinew

To serve your turn long after they are gone,

And so hold on when there is nothing in you

Except the Will which says to them: "Hold on!"

If you can talk with crowds and keep your virtue,
Or walk with Kings—nor lose the common touch,
If neither foes nor loving friends can hurt you,
If all men count with you, but none too much;
If you can fill the unforgiving minute
With sixty seconds' worth of distance run,
Yours is the Earth and everything that's in it,
And—which is more—you'll be a Man, my son!

~ Rudyard Kipling

Chapter Summary: Part 1

1. It is only when we become **aware** that there is a field of reality within us—that holds the wisdom of health—and that we have the ability to choose to align our lives with this wisdom, does the ability to create health in our experience become possible.

2. It is only when we reclaim responsibility for our thoughts and ideas that we create the security required to stop engaging in imbalanced and conflicted perceptions, and create space to find answers to the fundamental question: "*What is the healthy course of action?*"

3. It is only when we stop taking life personally and learn to engage with others with equanimity that we reclaim our **power**. This power allows us to use our emotions to add color to our life—rather than using them as weapons—and create a foundation for healthy relationships.

4. It is when we strike balance between the left side of our mind—the side that is responsible for logical thought—and the right brain, which is responsible for creative thought, that we become leaders in our own lives. We gain the ability to envision a healthy life and execute action around that vision. **We balance the hemispheres of our own mind.**

5. It is only when we learn the art of **Emotional Alchemy**—that enables us to transcend anxiety and hurt and create confidence and well-being from within—we find our ability to create

happiness from within, and bring joy to our life.

6. It is only when we discover our own
    Uniqueness—or a sense of purpose in this world
    that arises from within us—that we are given the
    ability to embody our own independence in the
    physical world and create a foundation for
    interdependent relationships.

7. The first six principles of health combine to
    create the **Independent** core required to create
    life in a healthy manner. It can be seen as the
    masculine half of the health spectrum.

PRINCIPLE 7
Balancing Ethics and Worldliness to Create Mutually Beneficial Relationships:
THE TRIPLE-WIN EFFECT

"Ships are safest in the harbor; but that's not what ships were built for."

~ Grant M. Bright

The Young Grasshopper

Once upon a time there was a young grasshopper who loved to play his violin in a beautiful, lush meadow on warm spring days. Nearby the meadow was a large ant hill from which ants would go out each day and gather food to store for the snowy, winter months.

Every morning, three ants would leave the ant hill for their food-gathering ritual. As they passed the grasshopper, immersed in his musical whimsical ways, the first ant—who was a soldier of the ant hill—would scoff at his antics.

"Why do you waste your time playing music when you should be gathering food for winter?" he asked. The grasshopper, however, was too consumed by his passion and did not listen. He just continued to play.

The second ant was young. This was his first spring, and he wanted to listen to the music that mesmerized him with its beauty, but not wanting to be reprimanded by the first ant, he hurried on to find food, saying nothing.

The third ant was elderly. He had seen many seasons come and go, and stopped to listen to the grasshopper's haunting music, before thanking him for making his job a little more meaningful. He then continued on his way.

For the whole of spring and summer, the three ants carried out their food-gathering mission. When the autumn leaves began to fall from the trees and the weather began to turn cold, and the mornings frosty, the ant hill was prepared for the winter.

It was a chilly autumn day when the three ants were returning with the day's food portions to the ant hill. It was the very last day before they would settle into the ant hill for a long, cold winter. They had prepared well, and all was ready. As they were reaching the ant hill they came across the young grasshopper. He was sad. His violin lay silent by his side.

"Why are you not playing today?" asked the young ant.

"It is cold," answered the grasshopper in a sad and forlorn voice. "Food is getting hard to find and I have nowhere to stay for the winter."

The young ant felt pity for his plight. "Maybe you can stay with us in the ant hill for the winter? We could give you food and shelter," he said looking to the soldier ant for guidance.

The soldier scoffed. "I told him in spring he should not waste his time playing music and should work like us to prepare for winter. Yet he did not listen! Now you would have him eat the food we worked so hard for? How many grasshoppers would you have us feed before we all starve?" Both the grasshopper and the young ant looked down in shame.

The young ant thought he was right, but in his heart he still wanted to help the grasshopper.

As they were about to continue on to their hill, the elder ant came forward and spoke: "Grasshopper, you have been playing your violin all summer, creating ever more beautiful music. It has been a joy to listen to your art, even if only for brief moments. Our Queen loves music and I know the ants would find it enjoyable to listen to some lighthearted melodies through the dreary days of winter. Why don't you come play for us and we provide you with food and shelter for the winter in exchange? All of us will benefit."

The grasshopper looked up with hope in his eyes. "I would love to!" he chirped. The young ant was happy that the grasshopper was saved from certain death, and although the soldier ant grumbled about how he "told him so", he knew that the elder ant was right.

The deal was struck. The three ants and the grasshopper returned to the ant hill talking about the exciting concerts the grasshopper would perform.

That winter was the the coldest and wettest on record. Yet deep below the earth, in the heart of the ant hill, everyone was enjoying themselves. All the ants were warmed by the sweet music that floated from the violin of the grasshopper, who had become a master from his daily practice throughout the summer. Together they lived happily until spring when the warm weather returned and the plants began to bloom once more.

The wisdom of the elder ant had made all the difference and made everyone's lives a little warmer and richer.

Finding a Path Beyond Conflict

I remember times when I was younger and used to get my way most of the time. Being fairly smart, I would devise clever arguments as to why my opinion was right—be it grand ideas about how to live one's life, to simple ideas of where we were going eat out that day. I argued passionately for my truth. At the time it was kind of fun bending people's wills to mine, and feeling like I was the smartest in the room. I didn't always succeed, but more often than not I would win the battle of the ego.

After some time I noticed people started to resent it, resulting in arguments and some of my friendships were slowly undermined. After one particularly heavy argument, I started to do some soul searching and realized the selfish nature of what I was doing. My conscience had caught up with me.

I decided to become more "spiritual" in my approach— to be selfless more often, and to let other people "win" in matters of opinion. I began to let others make decisions, even if I did not particularly agree. Yet after awhile, I noticed myself becoming resentful. I was slowly turning into someone I was not. Other people started to lose respect, seeing me as a "pushover". This frustrated me to no end.

Didn't they see I was trying to be on their side by letting them win?

I felt stuck between being Mr. Egotistical and Mr. Nice Guy. I knew these personas were not who I was deep down, but I could not see a way out. After flip-flopping from one position to the other, and many frustrating experiences, I had an epiphany, and stumbled upon a new way of seeing the problem. I realized a new way of seeing life.

My study of the human body helped me realize that life, in its essence, is neither nice nor egotistical.

As I studied cells—the basic units of life—a curious question arose:

> — *How do a trillion individual cells that make up a human body live in harmony with each other?*

It was this question that grounded my insight of this health principle into physical reality.

Healthy cells choose scenarios that benefit both themselves and others in turn. They also choose pathways that benefit the body as a whole. With this understanding, I suddenly saw a window onto a path in the center of my experience:

> I wanted *"A"* and the other person wanted *"B"*, but there had to exist a *"C"* that we both wanted. *"C"* was something that not only benefited both of us, but also the society or community in which we live.

My eyes opened and my insight into the nature of health deepened. I began to recognize "C" more often, which increased the harmony in my relationships. Conflict is still a part of my life at times, but it is far less frequent than it ever was. Aligning with this principle of health brings more harmony to one's relationships, and embracing it in my life has brought much joy.

The Triple-Win Effect

The first six principles of health create a strong, independent core inside one's self that allows us to find and express the unique purpose we each bring to the world. These principles enable us to unearth our **meaning** from within, and create the stability needed to remain mindful of the internal **balance** required to create a healthy foundation for our lives. They ready us to relate to life and external relationships in a cooperative and constructive manner so that **harmony** can prevail in our lives.

The seventh principle sets the foundation for the creation of harmonious relationships. It describes the most fundamental balancing dynamic between the individual elements of life that health derives from: **Ethics and Worldliness**.

Ethics, as I use the word, simply implies the consideration of others and the greater good of a whole living system, including the views, needs, desires, and welfare of all beings within that system.

Worldliness refers to the courage to promote one's own views, beliefs, needs, and welfare, without the need to force it onto other people.

Striking the balance between ethics and worldliness
is acting in ways that are healthy for us, for others,
and for the system as a whole.

In her book *Triple Win*, the entrepreneur Darshana Ubl, introduces an idea that business becomes most successful when it serves oneself, others, and society as a whole. Companies that are structured on this "Triple Win" identity succeed because they nurture not only their own interest, but the interest of their employees, their customers, and the natural and social environment upon which humans depend. This ideal also holds true because it is founded on a principle of health.

In healthy living organisms, this relationship of mutual benefit is always observed. Healthy cells making up the "individuals" of a physical body always seek to benefit themselves, other cells, as well as the whole body. This kind of identity transcends the conflicts of Perceptional Reality. It enables sustainable growth and is a foundation for harmonious creation within a living system.

The **Triple-Win** principle arises when we become aware of its presence as an intelligence intrinsic to who we are as living organisms, and when we set our intention to apply its principle in our own lives.

Tuning Into Health

All of the principles of health are already operating within us. After all, we are life and health is our nature. The principles are waiting for us to tune in to their reality and make it our own.

Vitality can be thought of as a frequency playing the 12 Priciples of Health. Just like on a radio station, we tune in to a particular frequency to hear a song—so it is with health. When we tune in to Vitality, the principles of health can express themselves through us.

However, to activate its potential, we have to let go of— or tune out of—the perceptional frequency that may be playing us!

The frequency that tells us that life is about getting our own way at the expense of others, the frequency that does not see life as interconnected—this frequency has to go.

Achieving this requires a strong, stable, considerate, and creative core, grounded in our own independence. Without it, we will seek the approval of others by giving in to their desires, and without considering our own well-being. Or we may think we need to get our own way to feel good about ourselves at the expense of others.

The grounding of independence created by the first six principles allows a person to become open to other people's views and influences, and to listen with empathy without becoming subservient or sacrificing one's uniqueness and independence. It also enables a person to gain the courage to express their own world view without the need to force it upon others or compromise the freedom of others.

When we listen with empathy and speak truth with courage, we find a place that transforms positions from benefiting only us or another, into a new path that benefits both parties. We begin to ask not what perceptions we wish to uphold, but what is the healthy way forward in any given situation—for ourselves and for others.

To fully embrace this principle we have to realize that even though we are independent individuals seeking mutual benefit, there is a bigger picture to life that unites us. We are all in this together. In the dimension of Vitality, we are one, and the healthy pathway benefits everyone.

Once we embrace the Triple-Win principle—once we tune in to its reality—it can begin to be expressed in the way we relate to:

— *Our bodies via diet and exercise*
— *The way we create relationships with our family, friends, work colleagues, and business structures*
— *The environment through farming and mining practices*
— *Organizing economic systems upon which we have founded our society*
— *Our daily living*

Ultimately, we have to consider the way we as humans treat the animals and ecosystems on this planet. In the end, health is one, and we are in it together.

Striking a Balance

Without the independent core of stability created by embracing the first six principles, a person is often unable to strike this balance. They often overbalance into worldliness and defensiveness, like the soldier ant who was only interested in his own world view, with no consideration of the plight of others. Similarly, one can overbalance in ethics, like the young ant who would simply give without considering the needs of the whole ant hill.

The ability to listen with empathy, to consider the position of others and how it can relate harmoniously to one's own position—and that of the whole community—is the hallmark of this principle. When the balance is struck, like the elder ant in the story, a person gains the ability to hold both positions in their consideration and choose a path mutually beneficial to both parties, as well as the community. This path is the choice health takes, and thus creates healthy manifestations in living systems.

The balance between ethics and worldliness is thus mediated by certain values:

— *Respect of individual perspectives*
— *Empathetic listening*
— *Balanced consideration*
— *Clear communication*

From this standpoint, potentially conflicting ideas can be transformed into mutually beneficial relationships.

If a solution is not found, the ability to disagree and part without loss of respect or integrity is also possible. Sometimes we simply do not find a mutually beneficial path, and in such a case, agreeing to disagree is the only viable path. Yet when done in an honorable way, health does not have to be compromised.

The argument of whether to consider others first or one's self first has been pondered by humanity across the ages. We consider this argument as the polarity between selfishness, which is considered bad, and selflessness, which is considered good. In the world of health principles, the answer to this conflict becomes clear: It is healthy to do both at the same time.

Maturing From Independent to Interdependent

The union of these two polarities creates a third position that benefits both parties. We don't have to be good or bad—we just have to be real. This kind of relating with mutual benefit is a sign of relationship maturity.

Choosing to commit our lives to the principle of mutually beneficial relationships, our journey expands and we move from **independent** to experiencing life as **interdependent**.

Setting out on this journey there is no certainty as to what will be found, what challenges will be faced, and dangers that may arise. Just like the sailors of old who sailed out to discover new lands, a person requires a spirit of adventure, courage, a curiosity for discovery, and a passion for creativity to embark on such a journey. The Triple-Win principle becomes the compass that enables us to take this journey safely. It prevents us from becoming shipwrecked in the shores of perceptional conflict.

Relation-ships are safest when we stay in the harbor of Independence. Here, we know who we are and what we stand for. Yet that's not what relationships were built for.

Life is is a process of co-creation, and health requires us to set sail and work together with others. We seek pathways beyond conflict and to build experiences greater than the sum of the individuals involved. To do this, we have to set sail upon the great Ocean of Life. And as we sail deeper into the reality of life, we become aware that we are not alone—we too are part of the ocean. And in the ocean, harmony is flowing and guiding us from within. This awareness engages in us the next principle of health: the principle of Synergy.

PRINCIPLE 8
SYNERGY:
Connection

*"We are like islands in the sea, separated on the
surface but connected in the deep."*

~ William James

*"Every part of the earth is sacred to my people.
Every shining pine needle, every sandy shore,
every mist in the dark woods, every meadow, every
humming insect.
All are holy in the memory and experience of my people.*

*We know the sap which courses through the trees
as we know the blood that courses through our veins.
We are part of the earth and it is part of us.
The perfumed flowers are our sisters
The bear, the deer, the great eagle, these are our brothers.
The rocky crests, the dew on the meadow, the body heat of
the pony,
and man all belong to the same family.*

*This we know: The earth does not belong to man, man
belongs to the earth.
All things are connected like the blood that unites us all.
Man did not weave the web of life; he is merely a strand in
it.
Whatever he does to the web, he does to himself."*

*~ Excerpt from Chief Seattle's letter to the American
Government, 1854*

My Experience of Synergy

There were times in my life when I felt lonely and disconnected from life. As if I was on the outside looking in through a window, but unable to participate. It was not that I really was alone—I had a very loving family, good friends, and an active social life, but somehow I felt an invisible barrier between myself and life that I could not breach. I could not quite see how I belonged.

This disconnect caused an awkwardness in my relationships at times. It sparked a search for a distant something that I could not quite remember, yet something that whispered to my subconscious mind.

One day it found me, and the barriers came tumbling down.

When I experienced my epiphany, and then Vitality, I gained a sense of deep connection to life, as if awoken from slumber. My heart opened to what it really meant to be alive. This experience of **Synergy** was a mysterious experience, often associated with a sense of stillness and inner peace. From that place emanated a feeling of deep connection with the people around me and my environment—also a joy flowing from inside me. Suddenly I was stepping into an unseen ocean of experience that connected life. It felt like the "grace" of life had found me, because I wasn't doing anything to create it. It created within me a powerful feeling of gratitude and wonder.

I could be all alone, but I could never be lonely with its presence.

I was feeling, thinking, speaking, and acting in ways that harmonized with the people around me—we were part of a web of life, a greater, invisible whole, that influenced our paradigm, and how we interacted with each other and the world. I guess some people call it the dawning of the experience of **love**. Some call it the *Grace of God*. I call it **Synergy**.

Synergy is the constructive union of individual elements of life.

It is the principle that enables the interaction of two or more elements of life, in a manner that produces a combined reality greater than the sum of their separate realities.

With synergy, I was transcending conflict. I felt alive with great purpose, balanced, and in tune with life. It was the place from which harmony flowed. These moments have come and gone, yet the experience—even for short periods—is the realization that life is far more connected, beautiful, and mysterious than the logical mind would ever care to admit.

Synergy describes the ability to experience the harmony and unity that flows through all living systems and underpins the creative potential of life. It is a key ingredient in one's ability to create a healthy life. Within ourselves lies the ability to connect with the experience of this creative intelligence, to experience being part of a greater whole.

Although we are islands in the great ocean of life, deep down, we are connected.

Unlocking Creative Potential

Harmonious relationships that spring from Synergy transcend perceptional, polarized positions. They create a movement of expression that is mutually beneficial and unified.

Where the Triple-Win principle allows us to logically structure life in mutually beneficial ways, synergy enables us to emotionally experience being part of this co-creative expression. It enables us to "see" beyond the perception of separation. Synergy does not operate through reason, but through direct experience, and it fuels a person's creativity.

Synergy is not a static reality. It is dynamic, flowing, and adapts to life. It takes one on a journey of co-creation, to a creative potential that enables us to move out of one's own Perceptional Reality.

Synergy is founded on the previous seven principles. As the clouds of Perceptional Reality diminish on our journey towards Vitality, the light of synergy burns more brightly. It enables us to feel safe to open up to the uncertainty of life since we are no longer alone—we are a part of a greater reality.

In Perceptional Reality, we build concrete, dualistic positions that stand on the emotions of fear, anger, desire, and pride, leading to conflicted relationships as we fight to defend our perceptions. The unity of life disappears behind an illusionary veil of separation. Synergy, however, transcends this experience. The illusion recedes and allows us to see behind the veil; to wake up to a greater reality of which we are a part. We can see that the nature of life is not conflict, but driven by health.

Applying Synergy

Within our bodies, this principle is a fundamental key that enables cells to create a healthy body. Together, billions of cells, many of which hold different meanings and express very different actions of behavior, create a living organism that behaves as a unified whole.

This synergistic principle is mediated by the nervous system, and allows the cells to evolve the body so that it can grow, mature, and adapt to its environment—to exist in a healthy manner.

As individuals, we can apply the principle of synergy to connect and form healthy family bonds, social structures, communities, nations. We realize we are all citizens of Earth and can seek ways to relate to the planet in a sustainable, healthy way.

Chief Seattle's letter to the American Government echoes the synergy his people saw as a key to relating to the land in a healthy manner: "This we know. The earth does not belong to man, man belongs to the earth ... Whatever he does ... he does to himself."

We are all part of a greater whole.

The experience of synergy ripples out into the way we see and think about our life. It enables us to value and respect the differences in others, to build upon the strengths of individuals and to compensate for weakness. Synergy does not strive to create equal value. It strives to see the unique value of every individual to enrich the social structure we live in. Everything already has an intrinsic value in itself.

Synergy takes our focus from the *content* of life to its **context**.

Synergy asks:

— *How does all this come together to create a healthy whole?*

The author Helen Keller once wrote:

"Alone we can do so little; together we can do so much."

Synergy empowers us all.

Synergy is magical because it is non-local, existing as a field of connection forging unseen bonds between individuals. When we begin to experience synergy we start to experience an increasing sense of freedom in our lives. As we shall discover from the next principle, freedom is found when one comes into alignment with the order of health.

PRINCIPLE 9
Balancing Freedom and Order:
Harmonious Creation

"For to be free is not merely to cast off one's chains, but to live in a way that respects and enhances the freedom of others."

~ Nelson Mandela

The Story of the Eagle and the Golden Bird

Once upon a time there lived an eagle who was free to fly wherever he pleased. He was the master of his own destiny, hunting high in the mountains. His life was filled with adventure.

One day he was flying over a village at the foot of the mountains, and saw a golden cage on the window sill of a large house. Inside the cage was the most beautiful bird he had ever seen. The bird sang a soft, beautiful melody.

The beauty of the bird and her enchanting voice mesmerized the eagle and he flew down for a closer look. Upon seeing the eagle, the golden bird was filled with awe. She had never seen another bird so courageous and free to fly into the mountains. The strength and freedom in his eyes took her breath away, and they fell in love at first sight.

Each day the eagle would fly to the window to woo the golden bird. "Come with me into the mountains. We shall be free together to fly wherever we wish and do whatever we want. We can have a life full of adventure!"

The golden bird was fascinated. "But is it safe?" she asked. "Don't you go hungry? Here in my cage it's not as free as what you speak, but I am fed every day and loved by the people who care for me. Why don't you move in? We can live happily together in the safety of the cage."

The eagle was captivated by the golden bird's beauty and grace. He was tempted by the safety and comfort of the cage. He conceded that at times he did go hungry, and danger was never too far away when stormy weather broke in the mountains—*but how could he forgo his FREEDOM?*

The golden bird was also tempted. The strength, courage, and freedom of the eagle, and his life of adventure was very attractive—*but how could she forgo the SECURITY and comfort of her golden cage?*

These two lovers, their hearts forever bound, yet neither willing to give up their lifestyle, were destined to be apart forever.

Yet high on rising currents, soaring above the mountains on calm summer sunsets, the eagle dreams of the golden bird that he loves so dearly.

And on autumn days, when the sun rises from the East, the golden bird gazes from her cage toward the mountains and sings of the freedom she once felt when the eagle was by her side.

No one knows what happened to either of them, yet the love story of the eagle and the golden bird echoes in the annals of time.

Finding My Balance between Order and Freedom

I used to love the idea of freedom, often feeling caged by the laws underpinning our social structures. I would often go on wild adventures to third-world countries where social order is much less guarded. I would tramp around the Himalayas, riding on bus rooftops to remote locations of exquisite beauty. I would hike alone up mighty peaks in the Andes just to feel the freedom of being in nature without restriction. I bungee-jumped and rafted in wild waters to taste the edges of freedom in freefall. Yet I always came back to an ordered, structured life, amidst the work of a medical doctor.

Few organizations are more structured than Western medical institutions. My heart and mind waged a battle: The mind wanted order, safety, and steady progress. The heart wanted to throw it all to the wind and fly in the embrace of freedom.

After years of this tug-of-war, I realized neither position was particularly healthy. The freedom of traveling the world without medical insurance and climbing unknown mountain peaks felt great, but as I pushed my luck I knew it would one day run out. And when it did, I suddenly realized the importance of order.

On the other hand, reason, progress, and safety were great. They established my career, kept me safe, but they stifled my imagination and creativity. After a few months, I felt a little empty inside, somewhat like a caged bird. I needed freedom or my heart would cry.

One day it dawned on me that the the more I tried to move into freedom, the more I attracted restrictive order. I realized that both extremes were one and the same—both as unhealthy as the other. This sparked the inquiry that somehow they had to balance each other—to synergize—to a healthy experience. "Freedom flowing through order" was not only the solution to the conflicts between my heart and mind, it also described the way healthy organisms grow.

Freedom Flowing Through Order

The principle of balancing order and freedom seems paradoxical. When we observe physical systems we see that as order increases they become more and more restricted in their ability to express freely. This phenomenon creates a seeming conflict between these polarities.

Take our social systems as an example: systems which are very ordered and controlled begin to erode people's freedoms. This imbalance makes people perceive those who create the order as bad, often making them rebel.

The rebellion for freedom is a common experience in human social history, yet it creates conflict that often leads to war and erodes the health of society.

When we look at social systems that are very free, or even anarchical, we see that this path also leads to conflict. The decay of social order often seems like everyone can do what they want and be free, yet it allows a tyrant to rise up, and gain power and control over others. The tyrant then creates laws to maintain their power leading to the loss of freedom. This creates conflict as people rebel against these laws. We see the pendulum has swung again, setting the scene for the next rebellion.

Both perceptional positions of complete order or complete freedom create Perceptional Reality and conflict. This creates an unending debate about whether we as humans should strive for order or freedom, and what the correct balance between the two seeming polarities should be. Indeed, the creation of democracy was invented to address this very problem, and has moved society closer to creating a healthy social system.

Liberal right-wing politics tends to promote individual freedoms, while the labor left-wing politics tends to promote order for the good of society as a whole, often at the expense of individual freedom. These polar opposites play against each other, and therefore democratic societies stay close to the balance point where a healthy position can be found. This kind of balancing act is closer to health, because it seeks balance between two opposing positions to avoid fighting. It seeks the balance point where healthy social systems spring from.

However, the principle of balancing order and freedom goes beyond simply switching between two opposing positions. At the balancing point, a synergistic unification has to take place for health to be created—where argument transforms into co-creation. Although our politics have yet to discover this place of synergy, we have to understand that the right-wing and left-wing belong to the same bird.

Increasing the Order of Health Increases Freedom

The order of health principles have a very unique property: in most systems, increasing order decreases freedom, but when it comes to health, the exact opposite is true. As one aligns with the principles of health they experience an increase in freedom.

— How does this happen?

When a living organism aligns their expression with the principles of health, it creates independent stability, mutually beneficial relationships, and harmony with its environment. As a result, it is often granted **freedom** to evolve synergistically with its own uniqueness, which reciprocates harmony created by the individual.

Yet it is the internal freedom of finding a sense of peace from within—even when we are physically restricted by Perceptional Reality—that is the true key to our freedom. This enables us to step out of perceptional experience and to be in a state of health, even when our external circumstances do not reflect that. We can be within the perceptional circumstance, but not be caught within its trappings.

If one is able to hold this "space" of Vitality, the external world also tends to shift. We begin to find doors where Perceptional Reality had only walls. By seeking to create relationships that benefit all, we create a set of circumstances where life begins to echo the Vitality and freedom we feel inside back to us in our physical reality.

*We find that life grants freedom, as long as we
approach it in a healthy manner.
Health is the gatekeeper of our experience of
freedom.*

Navigating the ocean of life, it is wise to pay heed to the lighthouses—the principles of health. Not because they are rules, not because we are subservient to them, but because they are beacons that illuminate a path to freedom.

The order of health is the foundation that allows us to be free. This is why Nelson Mandela noted that to be free is not merely to cast off one's chains, but to live in a way that respects and enhances the freedom of others. He realized that freedom is a collective idea, that we are all in this together.

At its heart, life is conspiring to grant us the freedom we seek. We are free to choose anything. It only asks that whatever we do, we do it in a healthy manner.

*Life seeks the well-being of all living things. So as
we dance within the context of our own lives, let us
dance to the rhythms and harmonies of health.*

The principles on which health stands are not perceptions. Their safety does not create a cage. Their freedom does not put us in harm's way. Quite the opposite, they enable us to unite with the eagle within us that longs for freedom as well as the golden bird that longs for stability and safety. In their synergy, through their love story, we have the ability to create a loving relationship to our lives that flies on the wings of harmonious creation.

PRINCIPLE 10
The Cycles of Life:
Creating Connection and Sustainable Evolution

*"It's the Circle of Life, and it moves us all.
Through despair and hope. Through faith and love.
'Til we find our place, on the path unwinding.
In the circle, the circle of life."*

~ The Lion King

*"The circle has healing power. In the circle, we are
all equal. There is no one in front of you and there is
no one behind you. No one is above you and no one
is below you. The Circle is Sacred because it is
designed to create Unity.*

*The hoop of life is also a circle. On this hoop there is
a place for every species, every race, every tree,
and every plant. It is this completeness of life that
must be respected in order to bring about health on
this planet."*

~ Lakota Wisdom

Discovering the Circle of Life

There was a time in my life when I hated endings, especially relationship endings that brought my heart so much grief. I would resist endings even if I knew that ending was the only course of action that made sense, and even when my resistance was causing an ever-increasing amount of emotional pain in my life—and too often, in the lives of others.

It was only later I realized my resistance to endings was creating a blockage in the natural cycles of my life. It was eroding harmony, my evolution, and therefore health in my relationship experiences.

At the time I didn't know I was thinking about it perceptionally:

> *"Relationship beginnings" were good and to be valued greatly, and "relationship endings" were bad and to be resisted at all cost.*

In equal measure to my resistance and dislike of endings, I loved new beginnings. I loved to explore new places, have new experiences, and new relationships. I loved the energy of the new.

In hindsight, it's kind of ironic I could not see the connection between these two seemingly opposite polarities. I could not see that one depended on the other. I could not see that they were simply different sides of the same coin. New beginnings required endings.

Eventually I saw that life operates in cycles that are natural and essential in the healthy evolution of living things.

When I first experienced Vitality, I suddenly saw the big picture of life and how all the pieces came together. It dawned on me that I was creating all the emotional pain in my life. I was responsible for the conflicts in my close relationships, I was blocking their natural flow.

> *I simply had to let go and allow life to flow in its natural rhythm. To Embrace the cycles of life. To Trust life.*

At first it took great courage, and it felt like my whole life was falling apart, like I was losing control, and would end up alone. Yet I found my independence and the courage to take such a risk. My "Winter of Solitude" sparked the principle of the **Cycles of Life** to start to flow in my life, and a "New Spring" was just beyond the horizon.

From the emptiness of endings, new beginnings emerged. New relationships formed, and within a relatively short space of time I found myself in a place I had only ever imagined. Life brought my way the relationships I had always dreamed to find. I found love because I allowed life to flow in its natural rhythm—because I embraced this important principle of health.

I realized I could trust the flow of life, that it was conspiring to build my life in a Vital manner. That within me—like within all living things—resides the source of Vitality that sparks health creation. When I accepted and embraced my deepest winter, I found within myself an enduring summer.

Reflecting on the Cycles of Life Within Our Experience

The principle of the **Cycles of Life**, captures the idea that life evolves itself in a healthy manner through cycles. This principle holds true for our bodies, our minds, social structures, and even the way the planet creates life on Earth.

> *Cycles are important in the connection and sustainable evolution of life.*

Life is created through cycles because that is the way seemingly independent living elements connect to each other. Cycles establish a flow of connection that enable harmony to be created within living systems. Cycles are a way of unifying life, and since life is a unified reality, cycles becomes a principle of our health creation.

Evolution of living organisms takes place from generation to generation, in a spiral manner of rejuvenation and renewal. However, this evolution must be sustainable, such that the great circle of life strikes a balance between life and death, and ensures sustainability of the living physical systems that exist within the boundaries of limited physical resources.

Let us look at how this principle is expressed in the various forms that make up our lives.

The Cycles of the Physical Body

Exploring our physical body, just like in the natural world, we see there are many cycles governing its dynamics. These cycles span seconds, minutes, hours and days—some even weeks, months, or years. All of them serve the key purpose to connect and unify the individual elements of life, in this case, the cells of the human body. These connections provide essential elements required for healthy life. They not only create connection but also drive growth and sustainable evolution of the body.

Let us explore three examples to appreciate how the cycles of life achieve these goals.

The Cardiovascular System

The beating heart, which engages in a never ending cycle of contraction and relaxation, pulses, on average, Seventy times a minute throughout a whole lifetime. This cyclical rhythm enables the heart to pump blood around our bodies via an intricate system of arteries, capillaries, and veins, in a constant flow that starts and finishes in the heart.

It takes about one minute for blood to complete its cyclical journey, and in this process all of the billions of individual cells of the body are supplied with the energy, nutrients, and oxygen they require to enact their unique purpose in a healthy manner.

The circulation system serves to unify the cellular elements of the body in a manner that is essential for the health of the body as a whole. This cycle is the heart of health for our physical bodies.

The Respiratory System

Cycling on an average of twelve times a minute, in a human adult, our breathing follows the steady rhythm of inspiration and expiration. It supplies the body with oxygen, which flows into red blood cells in the lungs and is then carried to all other cells in the body.

Oxygen is essential to life. It is the key ingredient that enables cells to create the energy they need to enact their unique purpose of keeping the body in a healthy state of existence. At the same time, during the respiration cycle, expiration from the body eliminates excess carbon dioxide, keeping the body at a healthy point of balance.

The cycle of the respiratory system is a great example of how the body creates balance of vital elements that benefits all the cells in the body, allowing for its natural health creation.

The Cell Cycle

There is a constant cyclical renewal of our body's cells—the basic units of physical life.

Cells are created through cellular division. They grow, specialize, and express their uniqueness. Then they divide again to form new cells, passing on their genetic material and apoptose, or die, in a healthy manner. Apoptosis becomes essential to make room for the next generation of cells. Over one year, ninety-nine percent of all cells in our body have been renewed in this way.

Our bodies grow and mature through the renewal of this cell cycle, which maintains a sustainable environment for health to prevail. It is fundamental in the evolution of a healthy human body.

Our bodies experience many other cycles:

> — *Hormonal cycles drive reproduction*
> — *Biochemical cycles govern metabolism*
> — *From birth to death, our lives are one large cycle ...*

It is beyond this book to describe all the cycles of the human body, but these examples illustrate why this principle is so fundamental to our health creation and the importance of understanding and aligning our lives to the natural cycles that govern healthy expression in our bodies.

Psychological Cycles: Mythological Cycles of the Mind

Within the context of our psyche, life also moves in cycles. It echoes the natural world.

Health moves with the harmony of seasons that enable a healthy psychological evolution to take place in our own experience.

Spring signals the birth of the new. This could be new ideas, a new endeavor of study, a new job. It may represent a new relationship, or a plan of travel. Whatever it be, it is a movement towards creation, an expression of our uniqueness. It is a time of inspiration and vision. A time of growth. The spark of evolution of who we are.

In summer, the vision of spring blooms in our physical reality. It is a time of action and connection to the world. We begin to practice our new job, or engage actively in a new area of study. Our plans are realized through application in the physical world. New relationships blossom into maturity. We take the holiday we have been planning and travel to the places we have longed to see.

Whatever it may be, summer signals the most active expression of any endeavor—the realization and expression of our plans and visions, and the constructive, creative connection with others and the world.

As the cycle turns, autumn signals the ending of our endeavor. A time for reflection. We have completed our studies, or work project. We have forged strong bonds in our relationships through a summer of experiences. We have returned home from our holidays with new memories. We have achieved our goals and dreams, and are rewarded with the satisfaction of our journey. It is now that we can look at what we have achieved, and enjoy the fruits of our labour.

It may be that our journey did not go to plan, or we have not achieved or experienced what we had hoped. Yet a cycle is ending. We cannot stay on holidays forever, and even close relationships do not experience an endless summer. The coming winter signals a time of letting go.

It is the winter of our experience that many people find so difficult to navigate, for it signals the end of endeavor. Yet it is now that we have the chance to reflect on our mistakes and give thanks for our successes—to evolve and grow a little wiser.

It is here where things reach an end point. Sometimes we lose our jobs, sometimes we finish a project and must start something new. It can also mean we have achieved what we came to achieve, and must take the next step and grow into something new and take on greater responsibility. Our holidays have ended, and it is time to rest and consolidate, waiting for spring to come with new inspiration and the start of a new adventure.

In our relationships winter can signal a time of difficulty. We have to face perceptions creating disharmony in our relationships. Sometimes this disharmony breaks the bonds of our relationships and we have to let go, move on, and learn from our mistakes. Other times, it gives us a chance to grow in our relationships. Realizing our perceptional errors, we can make changes in ourselves and deepen our bonds to others, evolving relationships to a deeper level.

Winter can signal a time of solitude. It is a time where we have to face ourselves, and grow in our independence.

When we do not resist the flow of life, if we find courage to let go of the past and accept our mistakes—to learn, evolve, and to let go—then every winter has an end.

Spring always comes, signaling a new birth, a new vision, a new dream, a new relationship waiting to be realized. A new spring in a relationship deepens our bonds, and helps us grow together in a relationship that has greater depth and understanding because of the winter it has endured. A new cycle of evolution has begun.

Embracing this psychological cycle of life, we find joy and flow in our lives. There is movement and evolution.

In the acceptance of the inspiration of spring, the passion and connection of summer, the reflections of autumn, and the silent solitude of winter, we find that at its heart, life conspires to aid us. It helps us to live our lives in a harmonious and connected manner. It drives our evolution and forms a foundation for our health creation.

Environmental Cycles: The Natural World

Just like our bodies and our minds, the health of the natural world is governed by great cycles that bring unity to life and create healthy sustainable evolution.

There are many cycles within nature, but let us consider three fundamental ones:

— *The annual cycle of the four seasons that drive evolution of nature*
— *The water cycle that unifies life through the essential element upon which all depend*
— *The day/night cycle that balances activity and rest, which living organisms require to create a healthy life*

Cycle of the Seasons

This very important cycle is created by the tilt of the earth spinning around the sun for a one-year period. This cycle holds the keys to the healthy evolution of our natural world.

Spring signals new life: the energy of giving birth and new beginnings. Trees and flowers bloom, and new generations of animals, birds, fish, and insects are born signaling a time of creation and growth.

Summer is a time of plenty: new life grows into adulthood and life is at its most vibrant. It is a time of vibrant creative activity, connection, and a fulfillment of the promise of spring.

Autumn, is a time of slowing down, reflection, and preparation for winter: many trees shed their leaves, and many animals gather food to store for winter.

Winter is often a time of decreased activity, hibernation, and rest: the natural world waits in introspection for a new cycle to begin.

Spring always comes, bringing with it the new generation of life, and the sparking of a new cycle of evolution of life on the planet.

Each cycle brings with it a set of experiences that help the natural world grow, connect, and evolve—a key principle of health for the natural world on our planet.

The Water Cycle

Water is the fundamental element upon which all life depends. Be it plant, animal, bird, or insect, the water cycle plays a crucial role in ensuring all living things have access to this fundamental element that is essential for the creation of a healthy ecosystem.

The water cycle describes the way water is distributed on the planet: the cycle starts when water evaporates from the oceans, lakes, and is transpired by plants into the air. It moves into the atmosphere, where it is cleaned, only to fall back to earth in the form of rain or snow, forming streams, lakes, and rivers upon which all plant and animal life depend.

Eventually, much of it makes its way back to the oceans, forming a home environment for marine life. From there, it is evaporated back into the atmosphere once again.

Without water life cannot exist. It is key to health. The water cycle enables its distribution to all living things. It forges a connection between all living things.

The Circadian Cycle of Day and Night

The day/night Circadian cycle is created by the revolution of the planet on its axis. This rhythm sets up the cycle of activity and rest for all of life on Earth. It affects gene expression, and is a fundamental force in the evolution of life.

All living things require a balance between activity and rest for healthy activity to occur. As humans, we require at least six hours of sleep a night to function in a healthy manner.

There are many other cycles in nature, like the tidal cycle driven by the moon, the carbon cycle, and the nitrogen cycle. All of these are important for a healthy ecosystem. It is beyond this book to go into the details of all the important cycles in nature, but from these key examples it becomes clear that cycles are a fundamental principle that drive health in living systems on a global scale.

Blockages of the Cycles of Life

When the cycles of life become blocked, and the flow of life stagnates, health starts to erode. The connection of life is broken, and sustainable evolution is eroded. We see this in our bodies, our minds, in societies, and in the world at large.

Let us look at how this occurs.

Blockages of the Cycles in the Physical Body

When the cycles of the human body are disrupted, health is eroded. One key example is seen when we consider the circulation system.

When the circulation of blood is blocked, unity is disrupted. Essential flow of nutrients and oxygen can't reach vital organ systems, leading to cell death and the manifestation of disease in those organs.

When this blockage happens in the arteries of the heart, we call it a heart attack.

When it occurs in the arteries of the brain, we call it a stroke.

These two disease processes are the first and third most common causes of morbidity and mortality in the Western world. Which underscores the fundamental importance the circulation cycle plays in the health of the body.

Blockages of the Cycles in Psychological Expression

Too often humans neglect to heed the wisdom of the cycles of life. We fall into the trap of believing that life is polarized. We become trapped in the "illusion" of Perceptional Reality; that having "more" is **good** and having "less" is **bad**, that beginnings are **great** and endings are **terrible**. This kind of thinking must stop if we are to find health within our psychological experience and the greater relationship with our planet.

When we block the cycles of life in our minds, we are unable to let go of situations that have come to a natural conclusion. It could be a relationship, a job, things we no longer need, or an outdated way of seeing life. Whatever the case may be, resisting change often leads to regret, fear, and anxiety that life has taken away something that we believe we need to be happy. Emotional suffering often results.

In my experience, I had to learn to embrace the cycles of life that enable me to grow, to learn, and to evolve.

When one door closes, a new door opens.

Life is mysterious, yet through its cycles it brings experiences that are healthy. But that often cannot be foreseen with our logical minds.

Life requires us to trust this process.

Blockages of the Cycles of Life in Our Social Expressions

Our societies, and indeed the planet Earth, is a "whole", just like our body. The human body can only hold a certain number of cells, whose synergies create a healthy human being. They all have to connect and support each other for health to prevail.

The planet can only sustain so many people, and so many life forms, to create healthy societies and living ecosystems. Humans have to create a sustainable relationship with each other and with the planet to create their lives in a healthy manner. All must be mindful of our interdependence with the natural world.

Yet, humans too often ignore this vital principle of life.

As a species, humans are deeply scripted in Perceptional Reality. Unfortunately, we have often adopted social systems that do not pay heed to the interconnected nature of life on the planet. Instead of creating societies that are sustainable, and connected with the natural ecosystems, we have adapted the perceptional idea that more is better and have established an economic system that has to grow forever in order to be deemed a success.

Instead of understanding that we are interdependent with the natural world, which has limited resources, we often think we are its masters, and see it in terms of limitless resources that can drive economic growth.

This Perceptional Reality is one of "bigger", "better", and "unlimited growth". This imbalanced and unsustainable identity, is consistent with the mythology of cancer, which leads to illness in any living organism. Just like cancer cells, humans have grown in an exponential manner over the past few centuries, and have been eroding the harmony of nature.

Because of our actions, we as a species, are eroding the health of the planet: causing global warming, and extinctions of animals and natural ecosystems. These erosions have not been seen since the last Ice Age, about thirteen thousand years ago.

Our inability to align with the healthy cycles of the natural world are the root cause of this global problem. If we continue in this way, we risk destroying our natural world, the same ecosystems which we depend on for our well-being.

Balancing Life and Death: Sustainability

To remain healthy, physical life has to be sustainable.

For every spring and summer of growth, there is an autumn and winter of passing away. This makes room for the next generation—the next spring.

As some wise, unknown person once poetically expressed: "God pours life into death, and death into life without spilling a drop."

The value of life is in the meaning of the journey, the expansion of our experience—not in the accumulation of stuff and endless physical growth.

In the perceptional world we see "death" as evil. Yet this is an error of perceptional thought. Death is not always unhealthy. The passing of the old so the new can live is a natural, healthy life process.

As one of the great writers on natural death, Elisabeth Kubler-Ross, stated:

> *"Watching a peaceful death of a human*
> *reminds us of a falling star; one of a million*
> *lights in a vast sky that flares up for a brief*

moment only to disappear into the endless
sky forever ..."

Perhaps this poetic reflection on natural death captures the health of this vital process.

Albert Einstein also personified this principle when he said:

"Our death is not an end if we can live on in
our children and the younger generation. For
they are us, our bodies are only wilted
leaves on the tree of life."

We have to embrace sustainable ways of relating to the planet if we are to find a healthy way of creating our societies.

Healthy Evolution

Because life evolves, the end of each cycle does not finish where it started. Instead it moves in a spiral fashion, growing in a creative manner along ever greater cycles of connection.

With the passing of each generation, and the start of the new, life becomes a little more vibrant, wise, and creative than it was. It becomes a little more elegant, more beautiful. The healthy evolution is one of experience and spirit.

We also experience this in our lives—within the cycles of our mythological experience. When we embrace the cycles of life, each cycle moves us in an ever-widening arc of inclusion of life. We experience our lives as an aspect of a unified whole.

In the end, when we pass, when our lives come to a conclusion, we realize that life itself does not end. Just like our physical bodies pass to rejoin the earth, our souls return to the ocean of Vitality from which life arises.

Having embraced the principles thus far, we are well on the way of creating a healthy lifestyle. Yet the world of conflict and perceptional dysfunction has to be acknowledged. Humans have been caught in this way of seeing the world for a very long time, and there is a strong "gravitational pull" built up within us to keep us trapped in perceptional dualistic thinking and feeling. Therefore, the eleventh principle of health is our ability to "Make a Stand". It gives us the strength to willingly choose health over perception in our experience.

PRINCIPLE 11
Relating to Perceptional Reality:
Make A Stand

*"Darkness cannot drive out darkness: Only light
can do that.
Hate cannot drive out hate: Only love can do that."*

~ Martin Luther King Jnr

Humans are deeply scripted in the paradigm of Perceptional Reality. Too often conflict has become the normal way of relating to each other.

It manifests as internal conflict within the relationship experience we have with ourselves, and which we project out into the world. It also manifests as outward conflict when we interact with people who project antagonism towards us.

The principle of "Making a Stand", describes how we can begin to relate to the world of perception in a healthy manner.

Making a Stand Within: Integration of Internal Conflict

*"The secret of change is to focus all of your energy,
not on fighting the old, but on building the new."*

~ Dan Millman, Way of the Peaceful Warrior

An Old Cherokee Tale

One evening an old Cherokee told his grandson about the internal battle of people. He said:

"My son, there is a battle that goes on inside every person. It is between two "wolves" that live inside us all.

One is evil. It is angry, jealous, and fearful. It regrets, is greedy, arrogant, full of self-pity, and guilt. It is resentful, lies, has false pride, and thinks it is superior.

The other is good. It is joyful and at peace with itself. It loves, hopes, and lives with serenity. It understands humility, kindness, benevolence, and empathy. It is generous, tells the truth, and has compassion and faith."

The grandson thought about it for a minute and then asked his grandfather:
"Which wolf wins?"
The old Cherokee replied,
"The one you feed."

Learning the Wisdom of Making My Stand

There were times when my past haunted me. I had made mistakes, hurt people emotionally, hurt myself emotionally, and made poor choices. At these times, when my perceptional past arose within me, I always felt emotional pain and anger well up in my heart, as I was being moved to conflict. My thoughts started to polarize, projecting blame onto others, or myself. I slipped back into a perceptional way of seeing and reacting.

It was at these times that I had to remind myself the most to stand my ground. To stop feeding the perceptional realities that provided fuel to the fire of conflicted relationships. I had to observe the pain as it moved through me—let it flow—knowing it was not the real expression of who I was. It was no longer who I choose to be.

I steadied my will and turned my thoughts and actions towards what I knew was congruent with health. If I did not engage with it, the Perceptional Reality I was experiencing would move on and disappear from my experience. It was in this process that I found a sense of acceptance of who I was, and my past that I could not change.

It made me realize that when I had enough humility to accept the undesirable realities inside myself—yet not engage them—I gained the ability to understand them and let them go. I became free to shift my focus to building a new identity and reality.

This process took courage. The pain was intense at times. It is not easy to look at your own darkness, and accept it, without projecting it outwards, without blaming others, or trying to escape it using any means. It is to take responsibility for your own emotional and psychological state.

As I stood my ground, I realized that the pain often made conscious what I had not been able to see about myself. It was a message that my life was not on a healthy path. It revealed the aspects of myself that needed to change—those that needed to come to the light of my awareness so I could understand them—and let them dissolve and be replaced with a healthy expression.

If I failed to do this, continuing to resist the conflicted perceptions, or projecting them into my relationships, they seemed to find a way to persist in my psyche and experience. They only fueled the never-ending conflict of Perceptional Reality.

Making a Stand became a path towards my growth, enabling me to expedite the journey towards my health creation. As I made my stand, I found I could maintain my balance while creating my life in a healthy manner. This process is ongoing and I must make my stand when internal conflict arises within me, but now the conflicts are more fleeting, passing more quickly. I no longer feel like a captive of my Perceptional Reality.

Making a Stand Within

The principle of Making a Stand on the inside means choosing an identity, and making life choices that are congruent with health. It means being able to accept, reflect on, and say "No" to any identity that is perceptional and founded in conflict.

The movement towards conflict is born out of a polarized identity—a core belief that there is a battle between good and evil, or a world of winners and losers. When this identity is projected into our world it seeks enemies to blame and judge. It is quick to anger, sometimes turning the judgement and blame onto oneself and projecting the conflict inwards. It always believes that the perceived enemy has to be defeated or that one has to become a winner for health to prevail.

Maybe we begin to believe that Muslims are bad. Maybe it's the power-hungry Westerners. Perhaps women are the source of temptation and evil—after all, didn't Eve eat the apple from the "Tree of Temptation"? Then again it could be men—haven't they suppressed women's rights for hundreds of years? Maybe it's people of color who cause social problems, or perhaps the white people who are controlling the system for their own benefit?

Sometimes we turn these judgement on ourselves: maybe we are the problem that is causing all our suffering and the suffering of those around us. Unable to forgive our mistakes or the mistakes of others we become depressed and lose hope, or become angry and lash out at a perceived enemy to create more conflict.

Perhaps we believe we need to battle to gain more, so that we can say we are a winner, thinking that will solve all our problems. But in our journey we create conflicts as we step on others to rise to the top, finding ourselves in an increasingly hostile experience, becoming lost in the swamps of Perceptional Reality. This is not the path to health.

Looking at global politics and social problems in the world today, we can see how we are trying to solve problems through perceptional ways of thinking and that this is causing so much conflict and erosion of health in the social interaction of the world today.

This "wolf" of perceptional identity lives within us all, and if we feed it, it grows in strength and power. Yet as the old Cherokee parable implies, if we do not feed it, we take away its power, and become free to to choose a new identity.

A Question of Identity

When we make a stand, we acknowledge that the real battle is not between good and bad. It's not about winning or losing. Rather, it is between a Perceptional Reality founded on duality and health, which transcends duality and creates a harmonious relationship between all of life. Interestingly, as we become increasingly aligned with the principles of health, it becomes clear that there really is no battle at all. The idea that there is a conflict between these two supposed opposites is also an illusion. Instead it is simply a matter of choice.

As we choose health, we begin to see the fears, hurts, and pains of the past that we felt were inflicted by our perceived enemy, as the very same fears, hurts, and pains that others feel were inflicted by us. We are all in this together.

Jesus famously illuminated this idea, when he spoke to the crowd: "He who has never sinned, cast the first stone."

It is not a matter of causation, but one of identity.

With this insight we can begin to accept and forgive the pain of the past. Forgive not only others who we feel have done us wrong, but also ourselves. For it is clear, that all the pain was founded on a mistaken sense of identity. It was born of ignorance.

Choosing Health: Making a Stand In the Moment

Instead of fueling the cycle of perceptional conflict and suffering, we can make a stand: we can choose health from this moment forward. You see, this moment is really all we have. It's all we really ever had to make a difference in the way we create ourselves. From this moment our Identity is created.

We make a stand for who we are. We are life and health is our nature.

Although it seems that the chain of cause and effect cannot be escaped and the past is destined to haunt us forever, we cannot go back, we cannot change our past. In reality, every new morning, every moment, signals a new opportunity—an opportunity to make new choices about who we are and how we relate. Our focus is not battling the old, but creating the new.

Every single moment is the cutting edge of life, and karma does not exist. It is here that time falls away: the past is gone and the future is uncertain. We are given the opportunity to re-create our identity, and set sail towards our health creation. This is the hallmark of Making a Stand within, available to us in every moment we experience.

Making a Stand For Humanity

The hope of humanity lies in seeing through the illusion of Perceptional Reality, rejecting its expression, and embracing health. Thus comes to light the wisdom of Martin Luther King:

> "Hate cannot drive out hate, only love can
> do that."

The folly of trying to create health by force was also illuminated by Mahatma Gandhi who exclaimed:

> "An eye for an eye will only make the whole
> world blind."

As humanity, Perceptional Reality has blinded us. We have tried this path so many times, only to end up fighting wars and spreading suffering time and time again. It is time to choose a different path. A path to create ourselves and our societies in such a way that health may one day become a worldwide experience.

Making a Stand: External Expression

"Great warrior, hmm? Wars do not make one great."

~ Yoda – Star Wars

The Story of the Two Knights and the Blacksmith

Once upon a time there was a small kingdom ruled by a just King.

One summer, from the dark forest, not far from the city walls, a two-headed dragon was seen to emerge. One head breathed fire, and the other ice. The beast attacked the villages at the edges of the city and destroyed everything in its path.

Despite all the best efforts of the King's soldiers, none could stop the savage beast.

The King gathered his most senior advisors and they decided to send for help. Anyone who could slay the beast would be given the title of lord and a great reward.

Before a few days passed, a Red Knight rode boldly into the city gates on a mighty war horse. Whispers of a hero resounded throughout the city. He was brought before the King.

"I will rid your kingdom of this creature if you make me the most powerful lord and reward me with half your kingdom," commanded the Red Knight.

The King did not like the arrogance of this youthly stranger, but for the survival of his kingdom, he reluctantly agreed. The Red Knight rode out towards the dark forest followed by cheers from the people.

At the edge of the forest the two-headed beast appeared angry and seething with hatred. With a great roar, and fire and ice spilling forth from its heads, the beast charged at the knight.

Drawing his saber, the knight bellowed ferociously: "You shall die! To victory!"

They clashed and fought wildly. Fire hit the knight's shield, his saber flew in all directions. The Red Knight carved his way through the dragon's defenses and with a mighty effort he cut off the ice-breathing head. The dragon retreated with a roar of fear and anger back into the dark forest.

The Red Knight was an immediate hero. The king gave him half of the kingdom and as summer turned to autumn, the Red Knight became the most powerful Lord in the King's Court. Yet despite all his power and fame, he wanted more.

The Red Knight began a plot to topple the King so that he could rule the kingdom.

The King's advisors learned of the knight's plot and warned the King. They knew that unless the knight was stopped, his power lust would destroy the stability of the whole kingdom, and threaten their own positions.

The Red Knight was put on trial for planning treason, prosecuted, and banished.

On a cold winter's day, the Red Knight rode out alone on his horse to the cries of "Traitor!" from the people of the city. He yelled back in anger: "I will have my revenge!"

Yet he was never seen again.

Winter rolled into spring, and the wounded dragon had recovered in his cave deep in the heart of the dark forest. His severed head had regrown. The beast emerged again, breathing fire and ice, and terrorizing the villages of the kingdom.

The King sent out messengers to all the lands calling for help and promising a great reward.

Soon a White Knight rode into the city on a white steed. Whispers of a "savior" spread throughout the city.

"My King", spoke the White Knight, "I come from a distant land. Having heard the plight of your people, I seek no reward. I will destroy this evil beast for the good of the kingdom." The King was astounded by such a generous pledge.

As the White Knight rode towards the dark forest, he heard a mighty roar, and the angry beast with the two heads charged towards him. The White Knight, drew his mighty broadsword upon his white steed and bellowed: "For goodness I slay the evil beast!" and charged toward the dreaded beast.

Ice and fire flew from the heads of the dragon, yet a mighty swing of the knight's broadsword cut off the fire-breathing head. The dragon reeled with pain and defeat, and retreated back to the forest.

Impressed by the White Knight, the King said: "You shall have your reward and become a lord as promised". Yet the White Knight refused.

"I vanquished the evil beast in the name of good. I do not wish for anything," replied the Knight. "I will live with the monks in the cathedral."

The generosity and virtue of the Knight spread like wildfire through the city. The people had a savior. As summer rolled into autumn, he was glorified and exalted by the people. The White Knight was so idolized for his perfection that a rumour started that he should be heir to the throne.

The King's son learned that his power was threatened and began a plot against the White

Knight. He fabricated a story that the knight was using his popularity to create a coup against the King and take power for himself. Upon hearing this, the King tried and sentenced the White Knight for treason and he was banished.

On a cold winter's day, the White Knight rode out silently to the curses of the people who had not long before cheered for him as a savior. Now a broken-hearted man, he was never seen again.

Spring came again and the dragon's vigor was again renewing.

As summer came, he burst out of hiding and terrorized with a greater ferocity. For the third time, the King sent messengers to call for help, yet no one came.

Days passed into weeks and the King began to despair that no one would come save their kingdom. Just as all hope seemed lost, there was a stirring in the court. A young blacksmith, dressed in a black velvet vest was brought forward before the King.

"If you succeed in ridding us of the beast a great reward and half the kingdom will be yours," promised the King to the blacksmith, who smiled before quickly leaving the court and riding out of the city gates upon his black horse.

Near the dark forest, the blacksmith dismounted his horse. Drawing a spear that was strapped to the horse's side, he continued on foot towards the forest.

A terrible roar boomed from the forest as the two-headed monster bounded towards him, its eyes filled with hatred.

The blacksmith stopped, centered himself, and waited. The monster ran faster and faster toward him, spreading his wings and rearing up on hind legs. At this very moment the blacksmith thrust his spear at the exposed chest of the beast. The spear whistled through the air and dug deep into the heart of the beast.

The dragon roared, and defeated, it collapsed dead at the foot of the blacksmith.

After eyeing the beast with a cool stare, the blacksmith withdrew his spear. He walked back to his horse, and rode back to the city gates to the cheers of the people.

The blacksmith was brought before the King to receive his reward.

"I know nothing of being a lord, my King," said the blacksmith. "I will take the reward to start my own blacksmith shop and to build a home in our kingdom."

The King was taken aback by his refusal for status, but granted him his wish. By autumn he had many new friends, and stories of his wisdom and fairness had spread near and far.

By winter the blacksmith had been appointed an advisor to the King, and in the following spring he fell in love with a woman from the city and started a family. He had many adventures with his family, and fought many other beasts, yet that is another tale ...

For now, here ends the story of the two knights and the blacksmith.

Making a Stand Against a World of Conflict

My work as an emergency doctor presents me with ample opportunity to make a stand in my relationship to a world of conflict.

It is common to see people present to the emergency department in deep emotional conflict, and who are psychologically unwell. Some have deep internal anxiety and depression that drives them to want to end their life. Some present with thoughts of aggression and delusion driven by drugs, such as methamphetamines, that drive their aggressive behavior. Often they are brought in by police because they have lost their ability to control themselves.

As an emergency doctor I am obliged to keep them, and others in the community, "safe". Yet they often do not want this kind of help. They simply want to go home and end their life, or continue their expressions of aggression. Such is the extent of their psycho-emotional turmoil.

It is in these moments I find myself having to make a stand: to hold these people against their will to protect them from themselves, or to protect others from them. Sometimes we have to restrain and sedate them against their will to contain their deeply conflicted behavior. Yet it is never done from the position that they are bad people that need "defeating". They do not represent an evil in society.

We make a stand in the name of health, to keep them, and others safe, in the hope we can help them find their way back towards a healthy outlook. In the hope that in the future they may come to a balanced way of seeing the world and be freed from the deep perceptional imbalance of wanting to end their life or hurt others.

When we make a stand it's clear: there is no enemy out there. We strive to overcome ignorance, biological imbalance, psychological conflict. Making a Stand is saying "No" to perceptions that are not healthy without losing one's internal balance and harmony.

In accepting, and not judging the conflicted behavior of others, we become free to do what needs to be done, without losing awareness that conflict is not the path to health. We have simply gotten lost and forgotten our true nature for a little while.

Making a Stand: External Conflict

The outer battle is created by the expression of Perceptional Reality by others as they relate to us. In this case, Making a Stand involves us being able to stay balanced and engage the conflict with emotional equanimity. This prevents us from being pulled back into a perceptional way of seeing the world by the "gravity" conflict creates.

To do this, we have to refrain from judgement of the perceived aggressor and accept their expression, with the understanding that we all get caught up in Perceptional Reality at times. This does not mean we let ourselves or those close to us be abused. No. We do what needs to be done to protect our integrity and those around us.

When the dust settles, we remain clear that fighting is not who we are. We are not better for having fought. Victory is not found in winning battles, but rather through creating relationships where conflict is transcended. Making a Stand in this way gives us the "escape velocity" to avoid being pulled into the perceptional matrix and believing that winning the conflict is the answer to our problems.

In the story of the Two Knights and the Blacksmith, the Red Knight approached the battle with a sense of inflated ego, a pride that came before his fall. He felt the battle was what proved him a winner who deserved more than everyone else, something he was willing to take by force if necessary. Yet this Winner-Takes-All mentality is a trapping of Perceptional Reality, and leads to a deeply unhealthy spiral of conflict.

The White Knight approached the battle with the idea that he was fighting for good and striving to defeat an evil. Although one may say he was selfless, he was caught up in a binary polarity that attracted the manifestation of the opposite expression. He was betrayed by the people who felt threatened by his virtue and didn't want to lose their power.

The Blacksmith however made a stand with equanimity. He did what he needed to do to protect the integrity of the kingdom and returned to live his life in a manner built by healthy relationships. He knew that a healthy life was not built on the opinions of others—as being seen as a winner or being seen as good—but was forged through the power of connection and healthy relationships. It was the way he created his life that held the keys to the kingdom of his own life. This is the healthy way of Making a Stand.

Making a Stand: Psychological Reality

The principle of Making a Stand is akin to the integration of the *reptilian aspect* of one's mind. This most primitive aspect of the brain comprises the *basal ganglia* and *amygdala*, which are responsible for our instinctual behavior involved in aggression, dominance, and territoriality. When this aspect of the mind is seeing the world through Perceptional Reality, it will instinctively turn to a "win or lose" or "fight or flight" model, founded on anger and fear. When we try to reason with this experience we create paradigms of identity that are founded on a world that is good and evil.

When one integrates the reptilian aspect of the mind by becoming deeply founded in principles, it is akin to taming the wild animal inside of us. One can still use the animalistic instinct to protect one's own integrity and connect to others on a visceral level, but the mind can be transmuted from a destructive raw energy to a constructive synergistic one, aligned with the wisdom of health. The passion is maintained, but is channeled in a healthy manner. This kind of integration could be said to make a person one of noble character.

When we translate it through our logical mind, we begin to create an identity that is unified and founded on mutual benefit, rather than a winner or loser mentality.

Making a Stand: The Human Body

In our bodies, our cells also "Make a Stand" in upholding the integrity of our health. In the example of cells, this principle is upheld by the immune system. A very unique part of the human cellular community—the immune system—specializes in eliminating cells, such as bacteria and viruses, which are programmed to destroy the cells of the body for their own end without considering the health of the whole. It protects the integrity of the whole body, stops cellular fighting, and returns to a dormant state of co-active synergy with the body.

Humans Can Change Their Identity

Human beings are not merely cells. We are not like the beast in the story. We have the capacity to learn, to change, and to align ourselves with the principles of health.

Humans have the capacity to change their identity, to see through the illusions of Perceptional Reality, and create themselves in a healthy manner. As such, our destiny is not set and our character can be altered.

People who are deeply scripted in conflict and imbalance have the opportunity to find their way out of this matrix and reconnect to the Vitality that drives healthy expression. This is an identity common to us all. In this way, society can move slowly towards a world where fighting is no longer used as a tool to prove a winner or to prove who deserves the majority of the planet's resources. Fighting isn't needed to prove we are good or are defeating an evil. It does not solve the many social problems we are facing as a human race.

We realize that it is only in creating our lives in a healthy manner that leads to the creation of a healthy, peaceful society.

Sometimes we have to make a stand to preserve the integrity of life, but our focus has to remain on our health creation, for the cause and effect are one and the same.

Health is the only path to health.

The principle of Making a Stand is placed near the end of this book because a deep foundation in the realm of health principles is required to meet conflicting situations in a healthy manner. It is in a manner that will not throw us back into the perception of dualistic thinking. Yet understanding this alone is not enough. One has to translate what one knows back into our physical reality.

PRINCIPLE 12
Balancing Knowledge and Experience:
Translation Into the Physical

"To know but not to do, is yet not to know."

~ Stephen R. Covey

The Fisherman and the Businessman

An American businessman took a vacation to a small coastal Mexican village upon his doctor's orders. Unable to sleep after an urgent phone call from his office on the first morning, he walked out to the pier to clear his head. A small boat with a single fisherman had docked, and inside the boat were several large yellowfin tuna. The American complimented the Mexican on the quality of his fish.

"How long did it take you to catch them?" the American asked.

"Only a little while," the Mexican replied in surprisingly good English.

"Why don't you stay out longer and catch more fish?" the American asked.

"I have enough to support my family and give a few to friends," the Mexican said as he unloaded them into a basket.

"But ... what do you do with the rest of your time?"

The Mexican looked up and smiled.

"I sleep late, fish a little, play with my children, take a siesta with my wife, Julia, and stroll into the village each evening, where I sip wine and play guitar with my amigos. I have a full and busy life, señor."

The American laughed and stood tall.

"Sir, I'm a Harvard M.B.A. and I can help you. You should spend more time fishing, and with the proceeds buy a bigger boat. In no time, you could buy several boats with the increased haul. Eventually, you would have a fleet of fishing boats."

He continued:

"Instead of selling your catch to a middleman, you would sell directly to the consumers, eventually opening your own cannery. You would control the product, processing, and distribution. You would need to leave this small coastal fishing village, of course, and move to Mexico City, then to Los Angeles, and eventually to New York City, where you could run your expanded enterprise with proper management."

The Mexican fisherman asked:

"But, señor, how long will all this take?"

To which the American replied,

"15 to 20 years, 25 tops."

"But what then, señor?"

The American laughed and said:

"That's the best part. When the time is right, you would announce an IPO and sell your company stock to the public and become very rich. You would make millions."

"Millions, señor? Then what?"

"Then you would retire and move to a small coastal fishing village, where you would sleep late, fish a little, play with your kids, take a siesta with your wife, and stroll into the village in the evenings where you could sip wine and play your guitar with your amigos."

~ Unknown

Realizing that Knowledge Is Founded in Action

The idea that "to know and not to do, is yet not to know", became grounded for me when I began salsa dancing in my 20's. I have always enjoyed the creativity of the arts. It engaged my creative mind, which balanced the very logical mindset one has to have when engaged in Western medicine. Dancing is also a great place to meet beautiful women. It was a win-win scenario!

Learning dance, the idea that "life is not a piece of knowledge" dawned on me in earnest.

I absorbed the theory of the dance within a week or two, yet translating that knowledge into the physical was different. It did not matter to your dancing partner what you knew, unless you could make it real in that moment. Unless you could hear the music, tune in to the harmony, apply the steps in rhythm, and dance in complement, through space and through time. Knowledge had to become a living, breathing entity before I could claim I "knew" how to dance.

The same is true of health. It is not enough to know the 12 Principles of Health. One has to step out onto the stage of life, apply them, and dance them out within the context of daily life. We have to fall, falter, and step on people's toes to experience that we "know, yet we still do not know" in reality. Yet with practice, with patience, and dedication to translating health into who it is we are, it becomes possible to one day walk into a situation and bring your meaning with you—to stay balanced as you walk through the pathways of your life and harmonize naturally.

When I finally could enter that dance club, walk up to a beautiful woman, and dance for the duration of a song, improvising at times as we lost ourselves in the music and passionate fury of salsa, I realized I got it. The music stopped and we would both be smiling, for we had touched something real.

Translating the Understanding of Health into Our Lives

Translation of the intelligence of health into physical reality is the last principal of health.

Once we embrace the paradigm that creates health, we begin to flow meaning, balance, and harmony into various aspects of our lives:

— *The way we relate to and treat our bodies*
— *The way we approach our relationships and social interactions*
— *The way we structure our society*
— *The way we run our political and economic systems*
— *The way we as humans relate to the natural world, and the planet as a whole.*

Health is the path that transcends the conflicts and problems of Perceptional Reality on all levels of our lives.

Living organisms exist as a synergy of intelligence, energy, and matter. These three fundamental properties of life interact to create a healthy living organism. As such, health is not simply an idea. The intelligence of health must be animated through matter in space and time.

Mahatma Ghandi, the great Indian visionary, was once asked what he stood for. He answered:

"My life is my message."

So too, it is with health. One's life must become the health that one seeks. Our thoughts, emotions, and actions have to come into congruence with our physical reality.

Within our lives, this translation has to occur on the level of the cells and the mind. This then governs the way our bodies and social expressions are created.

Let's take a closer look at how the principles of health are embodied in cellular and psychological ways to bring these 12 principles together.

Cellular Reality: Creators of the Body

"The body is a community made up of its innumerable cells or inhabitants."

~ Thomas A. Edison

If cells—the fundamental units of life—were asked the question: "What is it that you stand for?" they would probably answer: "*My life is my message*". There is no separation between intelligence and living matter. Cells becomes animated along the pathways of their identity. Their fundamental intelligence drives their expression. Yet, each cell is an individual living entity.

Let us now look at a single cell from the perspective of the intelligence that allows it to create its health within its experience. Let us look at how it applies the principles to embody health as its identity.

Creating Healthy Cellular Identity

In order for a cell to be healthy it has to be connected to the field of Vitality from which health flows. The same field enables the principles of health to be encoded as an intellectual concept in our understanding. This is the **awareness** that sparks the cell to create in a healthy manner.

The cell membrane defines the cell's boundaries. The membrane is semipermeable, meaning it allows nutrients to enter in accord with its needs, while allowing toxins to leave. The cell chooses the reality that promotes its healthy function. This awareness to choose elements to maintain its own balance and reject elements that lead to imbalance is created by the intelligence of the cell membrane. It is its **security**.

The cell also has an innate ability to respond to life as it senses it in any given moment. It does not judge the many messages its outer cell membrane receives as good or bad. It simply aligns itself with health, and has the response-ability to meet the challenges of its environment to maintain its integrity in any given moment. This equanimity of function is its **power**.

From this secure position of clarity, the cell balances the leadership of creating the amino acids and other building blocks of matter it needs to function in its environment based on its function—and what the environment deems necessary—with the mechanical precision of its machinery that carries out the tasks. It has a balanced creative and logical construct. This is the cell **balancing its hemispheres**.

The cell now has the capacity to meet the challenges of its environment. Because it is founded in the present moment, and its focus is health, it automatically acts out of courage to do what needs to be done to maintain its integrity. As such, the cell maintains **confidence** in action. Knowing its deeper meaning as a unit of life—ever-connected to the whole and destined for a higher purpose—it is secure in its identity, which leads to a sense of **well-being**. Confidence and well-being creates the **emotional alchemy** that drives the **happiness of life**.

Each cell is an individual and has the unique ability to bring value to the body as a whole.

Some cells are liver cells that filter toxins from the body. Other cells are muscle cells that allow the body to move. Others, like kidney cells, filter chemicals to maintain chemical homeostasis. There are many a variety of cell types. No cell is better than another, for only together they create a human body. This **value** of each cell is its **uniqueness** that guides the cell's destiny.

The cell has now achieved **independence**. It has met the intelligence criterion to become a healthy member of the social structure called the human body. However, its journey is not done yet. For it is but one in a community of billions of other cells, all working together for a greater purpose. It has "matured" and is ready to engage in the greatest game of life, yet it needs to "understand" more in order to do so in a healthy manner.

A healthy cell is aware of Vitality, and thus understands that health within the greater context of the body depends on mutually beneficial relationships to every other cell in the community. As such the principle of interdependence leads it to serve itself—to maintain its own health—so it can grow to its highest potential. At the same time it seeks to serve other cells, so they too can maintain their health and reach their potential. Together, they serve the body as a whole, so the body stays healthy as a whole.

Heart cells focus on beating to circulate the blood that supplies nutrients to all other cells in the body. Brain cells focus on organizing the interaction of the whole in a balanced and harmonious manner. Lung cells focus on supplying oxygen to the body, which is key for the energy production in every cell, and so on. **This Triple-Win mentality** allows each cell to create a healthy community of cells that become the body.

Now that the platform of interdependence has been set, something magical occurs, which only life is capable of: the ability to relate to each other in a way that produces a combined effort that is greater than the sum of the parts. This process I call **Synergy**.

This unique gift of synergy is driven by a deeper intelligence of Vitality and creates a unification of identity. In essence, it creates a new living organism—an organism that can claim its own independence and uniqueness. Synergy allows cells to "feel" the unity of the whole and become part of something greater—part of the human body itself.

However, life is not static. Life evolves. Life grows. Life adapts to change. The healthy cell understands this too. As such, a cell is always ready to change: to change in a way that helps itself, and in turn other cells, to thrive. It changes without compromising the founding principles of health. This balance between evolution and stability is the balance between **order and freedom**.

Being rooted deeply in the principles of health becomes the greatest freedom. For health is the only way that life evolves in a free manner. This is called **Harmonious Creation**, and it drives the flow of healthy growth of living things.

Individual life does not grow forever. This kind of linear thinking is not congruent with health. Instead, a cell goes through a cycle of life that ensures sustainability of the living systems, and sparks life's intergenerational evolution.

A cell is created from other cells. It grows and differentiates, and executes its purpose. It synergises with life, creates from its uniqueness, makes its mark on reality, and then passes its knowledge to the next generation of cells through cell division, before it undergoes apoptosis (programed cell death), and returns back into the field of Vitality.

Within one year ninety-nine percent of the cells in our body have cycled and renewed themselves through this process. **The Cycle of Life** of the cell allows the body to grow in a sustainable manner and leads to evolution of life.

From this harmonious state of intelligence that has been created in adapting the principles of health, cells are given the platform to **"make a stand"** against elements of life that lack the ability to create themselves in a healthy manner. They preserve the integrity of heath for itself and for the whole.

This "all for one, and one for all" mentality is embodied in the immune system of the body. The immune system's job is to locate and eliminate cells and living things that are not aligned with the principles of health, and threaten the health of the body as a whole, such as pathogenic viruses and bacteria. When their job is done and the "threat" is no more, they return to live in harmony with the body as a whole.

As the cells embrace these principles in their own reality, as they **translate knowledge into experience**, they find they are not only understanding health, but they are becoming healthy. They are creating a body whose systems embody the Keys of Health. The organ systems of the body have meaning, are balanced, and create in a harmonious manner. They operate as one. Their life is their message, and it is held in the field of Vitality which has created it.

The embodiment of the 12 Principles of Health enable cells to construct the body in a meaningful, balanced, and harmonious manner. It is a manifestation of health in the physical form, arising from the healthy identity that cells have embraced in their expression.

It is beyond this book to discuss the minute details of how the cells use the 12 principles of health to relate to the physical elements of life and create organ systems that are structured in ways that embody the three Keys of Health. This however will be discussed in the second book of this series.

Translation of Health Principles Into Social Reality

"As above, so too below."

~ Maxim of the Hermetic

Let us now consider a human being as an individual unit of life. Let's see how the principles of health can be translated from an understanding in our minds to an expression in our social interactions and relationships to the natural world.

Just like the cell—a unit of life in a community of billions of cells forming the human body—the human being is a unit of life in a community of billions of living things that create a human society, and more broadly, the natural ecosystem of the planet.

Just like the cell, we as individuals begin the journey to health, through the awareness of Vitality. Because we are alive, we have within us the ability to become aware of this energetic reality that moves and organizes matter in a way that makes health possible. This awareness is open to everyone, because it emanates from life itself.

Let's take a quick journey through the 12 Principles of Health to see how they come together.

The **awareness** that we are not our thoughts, that we are not the scripting of our past, but rather, we are the innate knowing that creates them, gives us the freedom to choose how to lead our lives.

Having the wisdom to understand we can only control that which is within our own psycho-emotional boundary changes our focus from trying to control others and the world, to changing the way we interact with it. We change to shape our own character, to reflect what we are thinking, feeling, and how we are responding to the world.

The realization that we are able to make this choice for ourselves gives us the ability to say "No" to Perceptional Reality—which is fictitious, conflicting, and contradictory—and create the **security** we require to start our journey to embody a healthy lifestyle.

We realize that we can not only say "No" to paradigms that are unhealthy, but we can also stop reacting emotionally to unhealthy perceptions from others, and those generated from ourselves. We do not have to take life personally, nor do we have to react to emotions that no longer serve us. We do not have to attack others. We can simply observe the many visiting ideas and emotions and choose to accept only the ones that are health supporting, and let the others pass through.

We realize that emotions add color to life—they are not to be used as weapons. This equanimity of interaction is the **power** we require to become creative in our lives, instead of reactive.

As we gain understanding of what is healthy for our bodies and minds, through various channels of knowledge, we begin to align our lives around this knowledge.

The **creativity**, or leadership quality, generated by the right brain, has to be balanced by the **mechanisms** that make it possible, which are generated by the left brain.

We take action and create our lives to align with healthy lifestyles using our creative mind, and we organize and execute around this knowledge using our logical mind. We achieve this kind of control over our lives through the principle of **balancing our hemispheres**.

Having found the ability to create a healthy lifestyle, we use **emotional alchemy** to integrate our left and right hemispheres with our emotional mind (the limbic system) to create confidence and a sense of well-being. This generates happiness from the inside. This allows us to escape from any emotional subversion of other people who may want to hold us in dysfunctional perceptional patterns of life. It frees us to emotionally choose a healthy lifestyle by transcending addictive tendencies.

Having created foundations to become creative and proactive in our lives, we reflect deeply upon that which makes us passionate about life. We become free to follow our **uniqueness**—to express our personal meaning and bring value to others. We create personal purpose by this action, and contribute to society, thus bringing value to others.

We have reached **independence**. It is a state of maturity, so to speak. We have gained the ability to now choose healthy interdependent relationships within the context of the social structure in which we live.

We realize that social health is founded on the ability of its citizens to be independent and free to express themselves, but to do so in a manner that benefits others and the environment as a whole. This is achieved through empathetic listening, by balancing courage to express our needs and desires, and consideration for the needs and desires of others. It places us in a position to create a third pathway that benefits us, others, and the whole. It is an identity paradigm that begins to transcend the conflicts in our experience. This **Triple-Win** mentality creates the foundations of healthy interpersonal relationships.

The **Triple-Win** mentality allows us to use reason to structure our lives, yet we have to reach deeper and begin to feel part of a greater whole. The ability to do this activates **synergy** in our experience. This is the ability to naturally feel the emotional positions of others, and relate to them in a harmonious way with one's own position. This creates a whole that is more than the sum of its parts. It is the essence of how unification of life is created. We seek to meet our goals, not at the expense of others, but in a way that benefits others. Not only benefiting others, but benefiting the living system as a whole. As such, we transform from people of control, to people of influence. Yet our synergy has to extend beyond the scope of human societies. We have to reach out to consider the living systems of the whole planet—the same ecosystems upon which humanity depends for all our health.

As we embody our health creation, we experience increasing levels of freedom. For when we begin to live in a healthy manner, we begin to transcend conflict and are granted the freedom to express our uniqueness freely. This balance of **Order and Freedom** drives our harmonious creation.

As we grow in our own uniqueness, and our relationship to the world expands, we have to remain aware of the greater context of life. We honor the *Cycles of Life*, the understanding of which is crucial for the health of any living system. The cycles drive our growth and evolution. They help us grow in an ever-increasing arc of connection. They ensure sustainability of life. Embracing these cycles gives us a sense of grace within the impermanence of life.

Having embodied the principles of life thus far, we are ready to "**make a stand**". We choose health over conflicting perceptional paradigms. We choose to protect the integrity of life. Perceptional Reality is common in the human experience. Our ability to choose health, and say "No" to paradigms that erode health, must be embodied for our health creation to gain momentum.

Having embodied the principles of health, we are creating a new identity, through which we can flow this into the way we relate with the world. We apply it to the way we relate to our bodies, through diet and exercise, activity and rest. We apply it in the way we relate to our family, friends, and colleagues.

The principles can be applied to many aspects of our lives in a widening arc of connection. Beyond our personal lives, we have to consider the way we, as humans, create our financial systems, our governments, and global relationships to other nations. We must consider the way we approach gender and race differences. In essence, we have to consider the way we create our societies.

All of these can be re-framed from the paradigm of health to ensure we are creating our social structures in a healthy manner. All these expressions are founded on the identity of health that we embody through the 12 principles governing its expression.

The application of the principles of health that can create meaningful, balanced, and harmonious social systems is beyond the scope of this book. It will be discussed in the second book of this series.

Creating a Healthy World

"My goal in life is to leave behind a safe and healthy world for our children. Before I leave this world, I want to be satisfied that at least I tried. I know I can make a difference, even if it might only be a small one."

~ Maisie Shiell

Once our cells and minds align with the principles that govern health, they become able to create a healthy body and social structure that becomes our society. We, as a humanity, have a responsibility to flow health—not only with the arena of human experience—but in the world at large.

Never before in human history has humanity had so much influence on the living systems of planet Earth. Within the space of a handful of generations, we have grown from 1 billion people in 1804, to over 7 billion today. Humans live in all parts of the world and our influence on the natural world is vast. If our expressions remain unhealthy, we will upset the harmony and balance of nature.

In many ways, when scientists study the world, they already see this is starting to occur. Global warming, environmental destruction, extinction of many animal species, and topsoil erosion have been accelerating for several decades already. These are symptoms of the unbalanced and inharmonious way humanity is relating to the planet. They are symptoms of our Perceptional Reality eroding the health of our natural world. Yet, because we are part of nature, humanity will be affected by these changes. The planet is our home, and just like the cell depends on the body for its health, we too depend on the health of our planet.

Yet this can change, for life is change. Life is in constant evolution. We, as a species, have to change our identity for this to occur. As we embody the identity of health we can gain an increasing ability to construct our social systems to restore meaning, balance, and harmony—not only in our own lives, not only in the lives of human societies, but also on the planet as a whole. Because of our ability to change as humans, and our strong influence on the natural world, we have the great responsibility to ensure we are creating a healthy relationship to our planet and are not the cause of its demise.

If the health of the planet is to be maintained, our vision, too, must be broad and inclusive of all the living systems that share this remarkable planet on which we live. We have to ensure that we see the meaning of life. We have to ensure that we maintain the balance that life depends on, and strive to harmonize with all living creatures on our planet.

We have to ask ourselves: "*What is our meaning?*" in all this, rather than "*How can we get more?*". For meaning is the real currency of life.

Mythological Meaning

"We should give meaning to life, not wait for life to give us meaning."

~ Unknown

Do It Anyway

You can spend your whole life building. Something from nothing.

One storm can come and blow it all away ... Build it anyway.

You can chase a dream, that seems so out of reach,

and you know it might not ever come your way ... Dream it anyway.

This world's gone crazy, and it's hard to believe that

tomorrow will be better than today ... Believe it anyway.

You can love someone with all your heart, for all the right reasons,

and in a moment they choose to walk away ... Love them anyway.

You can pour your soul out singing a song you believe in,

that tomorrow they'll forget you ever sang ... Sing it anyway.

I Sing, I dream, I love, anyway ...

~ Martina McBride

Our journey into the intelligence of health is coming to its conclusion. Yet it's important to pause and reflect on the innate meaning that is created when one embraces the 12 principles that govern health. It is a meaning that always flows from within us into the world, and therefore cannot be destroyed by the trappings of Perceptional Reality.

The first six principles create our own **Independence**. This psycho-emotional independence founded the platform to express our own **Uniqueness** in the world. This sense of mission, of who we are, what we can give to the world is the **Masculine Meaning** that creates the inspiration to reach out and interact with the world in a constructive and creative manner.

We then evolved our understanding into the principles that drive the unification of life, creating the **Interdependent** reality through which life connects, harmonizes, grows, evolves, and protects its integrity. Embodying these principles creates the **Feminine Meaning** of loving relationships that create connection and joy in our experience, and that harmonize our lives, guiding our ability to grow and relate in an interconnected manner that is the hallmark of a healthy living system.

Together, when the masculine and feminine principles synergize, we see the free movement of a healthy individuation of life within the undeniable context of interconnection. We are unique and free in our own identity, yet we are forever engaged and connected to the reality of life, as it moves us all.

As we "square the circle" of these seemingly polar opposite ways of viewing life, we are able to transcend the unhealthy and conflicting world of Perceptional Reality. We begin to step into the river of **Vitality** that flows through life.

The awareness of Vitality brings with it a sense of being at **Peace** with the world in which we live. It constitutes the **Spiritual Meaning** that is the fountain from which health springs. This deeper meaning derives from our souls and is not something the mind can understand. It is something only the heart can see. It is an experience we step into. Our awareness of Vitality, that lies at the core of life, allows us to create our lives in a healthy manner.

So, let us next explore Vitality itself, so that we can find appreciation of this mysterious field from which health flows.

Chapter Summary: Part 2

1. Realizing that health is an interconnected reality, we stop engaging in win-lose or lose-win relationships. Instead, we begin to choose **Triple-Win**, or mutually beneficial relationships, that give us the ability to structure our relationships in a healthy manner.

2. To draw two or more things together in a harmonious fashion that creates more than the sum of their parts is **Synergy**. It is how health creates living things.

3. As we create increasing **order of health**, we begin to experience more **freedom** in our lives. We become free to express and create our lives in accordance to our vision of life.

4. When we become in tune with nature, and embrace the **Cycles of Life** that move us and pulse through all living things, we find the serenity that enables us to come to embrace life as it stands. This allows us to grow in our lives, and helps us accept the impermanence of life in a graceful manner.

5. When we embody the principles of health, we gain the ability to **make a stand**. To stand for health in our lives, saying "No" to Perceptional Reality that is incongruent with health. We make this stand from within and also on the outside as we protect life from destructive forces.

6. Principles 7-12 enable us to create our lives in an **Interdependent** manner. The ability to be **independent** and construct our relationships in

an **interdependent** manner, underscores our ability to create our lives in a healthy way.

7. When we embody the principles of health in our own experience, we begin to sense a deeper reality from which this intelligence springs. It is the experience of Vitality that transforms our lives, and gravitates us towards health.

Chapter 7

VITALITY

SECTION 1
WHAT IS VITALITY?

Integration of the Human Heart

"Someday, after mastering the winds, the waves, the tides, and gravity, we shall harness for God the energies of Love, and then, for a second time in the history of the world, man will have discovered fire."

~ Pierre Teilhard de Chardin

Vitality lies at the heart of the health creation journey. It describes how energy interacts with the world of matter and intelligence to create health.

The structured and defined world of organic matter, and the creative and unlimited world of intelligence and imagination, are bound together through an energetic bond. This bond, I term Vitality. In essence, it animates the principles of health through organic matter to create a healthy, vibrant, and creative living organism.

This chapter is described as the "Integration of the Human Heart", because it is the heart that has the capacity to receive and orchestrate this subtle energetic life force that underpins life—and thus health—in our conscious experience. This alchemy is felt as an expression in the heart, and as such, the harmonization of the heart with the body and mind becomes the key to the translation of the health principles into living reality.

Vitality is a non-local concept. The term "non-local" refers to the way that energy can occupy vast amounts of space at the same time and be transferred through long distances at great speeds. Technologically, this can be likened to mobile telephone waves, which can transfer intelligence, such as a person's speech, across to the other side of the planet within a matter of a second. Similarly, the intelligence of health is also present in a non-local manner, yet it is found everywhere, in every moment, where life is present. It resides within us, and all around us. It is more a matter of "tuning in" to its frequency that enables its physical manifestation.

> *Although this vital energy exists everywhere—and*
> *all the time—on this living planet, humans are not*
> *always aware of it.*

Often we are blinded by our Perceptional Reality that becomes our experience. When we stop engaging Perceptional Reality and start to feel the underlying reality of who we are in principle, we begin to experience the energy that creates the health interface between intelligence and matter. It creates a unique feeling in our hearts and bodies. The feeling is called Love, which seeks to create synergistic relationships that are in harmony with the principles of health.

Peace is the experience that arises when Vitality is present. In some traditions it has been termed the Peace of God, the source of true healing.

The Energetic Blueprint

*"Love is the affinity which links and draws together
the elements of the world …
Love, in fact, is the agent of Universal Synthesis."*

~ Pierre Teilhard de Chardin

Just as there is an innate intelligence that governs the health of living things—as described by the 12 Principles of Health—so too there is an energetic blueprint existing in a non-local manner that underpins the way matter is organized in a healthy way. This vital blueprint enables health intelligence to flow through matter.

Energy, as defined scientifically, is simply the capacity of a physical system to perform work, which is the movement of a force through a distance. As such, energy is what animates matter. It is what allows it to relate within space and time. There are many different forms of energy, as discovered by science, which are crucial to the functioning of a living organism.

- ***Kinetic energy*** *drives motion.*
- ***Potential energy*** *is energy stored in an object allowing it to move.*
- ***Elastic energy*** *is created by the stretching or deformation of solid objects.*
- ***Chemical energy*** *is stored in foods that living things can utilise for biological action.*
- ***Thermal energy*** *is the microscopic kinetic and potential energies of the random motions of particles making up matter, enabling living things to function.*
- ***Electromagnetic energy*** *has an oscillating electric and magnetic field that is emitted and absorbed by charged particles, and carried through space as* ***Radiant energy*** *in the form of light.*
- *There is* ***Sound energy***, *and there is* ***gravity***.

Yet no matter what energy the body uses to animate itself, they are all bound to the law that they cannot be created nor destroyed, but simply change form.

All of these energies act on living matter to animate it. Yet all of them can either harm or aid the health of a living organism.

So what determines which it will be?

This is where **Vitality** comes in.

Vitality is the subtle energetic field of intelligence that organizes all the energies that animate matter in a way that creates health in an organism. I term this **Vital Energy**.

It is *vital* because health depends on it. It is *vital* because it is the ring of energetic intelligence that binds them all.

Reflection in the Physical: The Hidden Storyteller

"We are not human beings having a spiritual experience; we are spiritual beings having a human experience."

~ Pierre Teilhard de Chardin

How does Vitality fit into the the health of a human being?

Imagine the body is like a story. There is a reason why humans love stories. It's because, in a way, we are one. Our body and our lives are a reflection of a story in which we live. Yet in this magical story, the three storytellers we discussed in earlier chapters are visible, while the fourth storyteller is hidden.

The First Storyteller: Cells

Uncovering the mystery of the body, science has discovered that at its core resides the DNA. This is the body's intelligence; like a library of books holding all the information of what your body is, and can become, as predetermined by one's genetic inheritance.

Each cell is the basic unit that holds the whole library. It is there that the book is read by intelligent proteins. Sections are copied, or translated, then made real by the power of transcription. Physical proteins are created to govern the functioning of the cells, which take on unique roles and create the structure of the body.

The Second Storyteller: Mind

The mind is the awareness of who we are as a human being. It allows us to look out into the world through the five senses, drawing meaning from what we perceive and act out in our lives. The mind decides who we are in relationship to the physical world created by the body and the world:

Who am I in relationship to my world, and how shall I relate to it?

This is the basis of our mythological identity driving our creative potential.

The mind has the capacity to embrace perceptions that are dualistic in nature and create imbalance, or see deeper into the dimension of principles that restore balance and gravitate us towards health. In part, it is inherited by what we are taught and the environment we find ourselves in. Yet, deeper, as we open our awareness to who we are in principle, we develop the ability to align our life with health—which is already present within us—and to choose to create this reality in our own lives.

The Third Storyteller: Environment

It is the collective intelligence of the bodies and minds of all living things that make up the ecosystems in which we live, and the social structures that humans have created. It includes non-living structures that form the environment in which we live. These collective identities also influence our perceptions of the world, and of who we are. They influence us because life is a unified reality and we are part of its creation.

The Hidden Storyteller: Vital Reality

Finally, we reach the hidden storyteller. Vital reality underpins and governs health in physical and psychological expression. This is where the mystery of life can be touched and where the identity of health resides.

It cannot be seen, yet its effects echo in the mind and body, and the world we live in.

When we look at our lives with our senses, we see the world in physical and psychological pieces; pieces that don't always come together in a way that make sense to us. It is only when we look with our hearts that we begin to see the flow of Vitality that creates healthy expression in our lives. We begin to see how the pieces relate and connect to create a healthy whole.

In the body, Vitality has the capacity to influence the intelligence of cellular mechanisms, which do the reading of the DNA. It coordinates what is read, translated, and transcripted into the physical, and how that physical expression is organized towards a healthy expression. It underpins physical health.

It also underscores the psychological structure of the mind, for Vitality helps us see the principles of health and enables us to understand our innate meaning, guides us to stay balanced, and creates harmony in our relationships. It allows us see how we relate to our world in a healthy manner.

Being non-local, it is present where life is present, so it flows through the ecosystems and social structures that create our environment. Its creative potential to flow health into living systems includes the whole planet, which too can be seen as one large, living, individuation of life.

Below the surface of observable reality, in the dimension of Vitality, the mind, body, and environment are one, suspended in a healthy energetic field underscoring life. It is the spring from where health flows forth into our physical reality, and begins to create itself in ourselves, and outwards in our environment, including the planet as a whole. It is the true identity of life to which we all belong.

From the view of Perceptional Reality, health is the end point of a healthy body and mind. From this vantage point we are like physical machines who have learned to think and have spiritual experiences of connection and unity—experiences that create the ideals of peace and love as the pinnacle of our experience. Health is the fantasy end point.

Observing the flow of Vitality emerging from within and flowing through living systems, we begin to see that Vitality is the energetic reality creating the healthy physical-intelligence matrix of living things. It underscores the reality from which health principles derive. Indeed, in the wise words of French philosopher and Jesuit priest, Pierre Teilhard de Chardin, we are spiritual beings having a human experience.

Health is real.
It is the distortion of perception that creates
disease—that is the fantasy.

Although **Vitality** is placed at the end of this book, in the reality of health, it comes first. It is the pillar upon which health stands.

Spontaneous Health Creation: Health Consciousness

"Every physiological and chemical transaction that
goes on in the human body is the result of a

> *blueprint of it within consciousness. All of them can*
> *be changed, by changing consciousness."*

> *~ David R. Hawkins. M.D., Ph.D*

Another way to describe Vitality is **Health Consciousness**.

Vitality is a morphogenic energy field—a field of energy that has an encoded intelligence in it—that carries the intelligence of health within it. As Vitality is the experience of the morphogenic energetic field underpinning healthy expression in living organisms, health consciousness is embodied in both physical and psychological forms.

> *The more aligned a physical being is with the*
> *Vitality of life, the greater its health.*

Vitality can be felt and this experience can be transferred. For example, when we walk into a room that is dominated by the field of consciousness of fear, it affects us. It gravitates us to feel it and embody its expression.

By the same principle, when you are around a person or a group of people whose expression is vital—or aligned with Vitality, the intelligence of health—it is easier to begin to experience that state also, and to embody its expression and express it in your life.

A person who is able to align with, and flow Vitality, is a Healer. They have a health creation effect on their own minds and body systems, and to some degree—because everything is connected—the mind and body systems of other people and living things.

Health creation is not a process of fixing disease, but of creating health—a state where disease is not present.

Because life is created and grows through cycles of renewal, every cycle holds the potential to leave behind perceptional expressions and embrace Vitality—to create a state of health in our experience.

When we begin to experience Vitality, the potential for spontaneous health creation is formed. There is a translation effect from the vital energetic layer to the cellular level. This is then translated into the physiological and biochemical levels, and so on, until it manifests as a physical expression in the body. This also occurs in the mind as the vital energetic field of consciousness begins to imprint upon our psyche the creation of new healthy thoughts and emotions that lead to healthy actions, creating a healthy social expression and experience.

Vitality arises spontaneously, for it is always present within us. Although spontaneous health creation seems like a miraculous event—because we can't see its causal origins—in reality, it's simply the way life operates. It is the external expression of our internal reality as living organisms.

Let's take a look at how we can connect to Vitality in our experience.

SECTION 2
CONNECTING TO THE WORLD OF VITALITY

Vital Interaction With the Physical World: Balanced Focus

"Obstacles are what you see when you take your mind off your focus."

~ John. Demartini

We connect with the field of Vitality as an experience in the present moment. As such, we require a balanced focus for our direct engagement with the content of the world to be healthy. A balanced focus enables a person to plan and execute a healthy lifestyle within the context of one's life. A balanced focus eliminates perceptional obstacles.

A balanced focus, speaking poetically, happens when time and space fall away, and what remains is only you and the object in focus. The balance point occurs in that very moment, between the future and the past.

— *What does this mean?*

When we focus "in the moment" on any particular thing, we bridge the space between the object of focus and ourselves. Space collapses and we create connection with our environment, enabling us to respond and relate directly to our circumstances as they arise.

When balanced focus is sustained, time collapses into an ever-changing present, and we experience a communion with the object of focus. We are connected and present in our relationship to our world. This timeless and spaceless experience constitutes vital focus, for it is the place where the flow of Vitality can be found.

A good metaphor can be seen in sport: when a great sportsperson gets into the "zone", their focus becomes balanced. Suddenly, their game becomes art. Their strokes become effortless, and everything seems simple and just right. This "effortless effort" is said to be the hallmark of a great player, and can only be achieved through this clarity of focus. Yet sport is only one example.

Balanced focus can be used to create a healthy lifestyle as it brings us into communion with our environment and allows us to transcend perceptional obstacles and translate our ideas and thoughts into direct action. It allows us to become creative in the way we live our lives.

Losing Balance

There are two ways in which we lose the balance of our focus, and distort it in a way that makes healthy interaction difficult.

The first way is when we lose our balance into the future. This is created when our desire to achieve a goal or outcome blocks our ability to see the situation clearly in the moment. The "desire" is a projection in time that pulls the mind away from the event into the fantasy. This creates psychological time and distracts a person from focusing on the task at hand, leading to error. A simple example is a game of tennis: when a player hits a tennis ball but their mind is already thinking of the outcome, it can distract them from the shot, and makes an error in hitting the ball more likely.

Similarly, on the other side, we overbalance into the past. This often occurs when we judge past events—projecting our past onto the present—also leading to error. In our tennis example, it would be like a tennis player miss-hitting a shot, and then becoming distracted by the idea they will miss again. Preoccupation with the past error makes them lose focus, and increases the chance of another error.

Obstacles are seen or created when we take our minds off our focus. This is done through the creation of psychological time.

As we learn to engage the world with balanced focus, we become increasingly able to interact effectively with the content of our lives. It is here, in the present moment—in the connection and communion with our world—where the flow of Vitality can be found.

Balanced focus takes us to where we can experience Vitality, but it is not enough.

Vital Awareness

The content of life only becomes healthy if it is engaged through a vital context. This context is created by engaging in Vital Awareness that connects us to the intelligence of health that holds the 12 principles.

If clarity of focus guides our ability to connect with the world and engage with it effectively, Vital Attention guides us on how we position ourselves to create a healthy relationship with the world that supports healthy expression.

Vital Interaction With the Metaphysical World: Vital Attention

"Where attention goes, energy flows."

~ Unknown

Vital Attention establishes a healthy context through which a person can engage with the world. It is created when we see the world through the prism of the 12 Principles of Health that underpin the intelligence of health creation.

Because health is already an innate state of living things, the ability to experience Vitality already exists within us. Connecting with it it is more a matter of aligning one's attention to its reality.

Our hearts have the capacity to feel the flow of Vitality. As such, having an open heart, or seeing life through the heart, can flow the vital experience through one's mind and body, and bring Vitality to life in our experience.

When our awareness opens to vital attention, we start to act in ways that bring benefit and growth to ourselves. We ensure our own **security**, **power**, **balance of mind**, **happiness**, and expression of our **uniqueness** are flowing within our life.

We also seek to promote ourselves in ways that create **mutual benefit for others**. Ways that create **synergistic relationships**, and connection and growth through the natural **cycles of life**. We seek to **protect life**. This order on which health is founded becomes an expression of our **freedom**.

Losing Vital Attention

Vital attention is lost, when, instead of seeing the world through the context of the principles of health, we see it through the context of a polarized perceptional matrix. When this occurs, we see life as a struggle. We see a world of winners and losers. A world of haves and have-nots. In this polarity we create a context founded on conflict that breaks up the unity of life, leaves us feeling isolated, and erodes our health creation.

Even if we have balanced focus and are engaging with the content of the world effectively, it will be of no use. If our context is unhealthy, we will simply be very effective at creating unhealthy situations in our lives.

> *There is no point running fast when you are on the wrong road.*

We have to engage both balanced focus and vital attention to create the experience of Vitality in our reality.

Balanced focus allows us to interact effectively with the content of our life. It creates connection and communion in the moment. Vital Attention enables us to "see" our life in a healthy manner as we interact with the content. It sets up a healthy context that infuses meaning, balance, and harmony into our lives. Through space and time, it sees the greater picture of how we are all connected to each other in the underlying unity of life.

Together, balanced focus and vital attention become the doorway through which we step into the flow of Vitality.

SECTION 3
THE EXPERIENCE OF VITALITY

Stepping Into the Flow of Vitality

*"Faith does not need to push the river because faith
is able to trust that there is a river. The river is
flowing. We are in it."*

~ Richard Rohr

We have looked at the nature of **Vitality**, what it is, and how it relates to our minds and bodies. We looked at the importance of **balanced focus** and **vital attention** in sparking its reality in our experience. Yet the question remains:

— *What do we experience when Vitality becomes present in our awareness?*

Vitality can be experienced as a flowing river of energy. It moves you in ways that creates health in your experience.

Vitality is non-local. It has awareness of all the pieces that make up your life.

Stepping into the flow of Vitality is an uplifting experience. It brings inspiration, motivation, vision, and passion. It brings serendipity—the experience of being at the right place at the right time—when seeming "coincidences" occur that are really orchestrations of a deeper intelligence connecting us all and seeking to support our health creation.

When Vitality is flowing freely, it's as if life has picked you up and is carrying you on a ride that seeks to build your dreams. This ride is not at the expense of others, but in support of building others' dreams alongside yours.

Stepping into the River of Vitality, we enter states of awareness that hold innate meaning. The experience guides us to balanced action in ourselves, in our relationships, and with our environment. Our actions begin to attract harmony to be created in our lives. As our experience of Vitality grows, it becomes the guiding light that whispers to us a way back home to our innate state of health.

The flow of Vitality is felt in the heart and carries the experience of love. Within the flow of its presence, our eyes open, and we see who it is we really are at our core. Like in the song, "Amazing Grace", we were once blind but now we see, and what we see is that we are okay. We are the health that we have been looking for. It is the grace of this flow of life that sets us free.

The Journey of Acceptance, Forgiveness, and Gratitude

"If I would have only one prayer, It would be thank you ..."

~ Master Eckhart

The journey towards the experience of Vitality is one of transcending the world of perception. **Acceptance**, **Forgiveness**, and **Gratitude** become experiential milestones on our journey.

Acceptance means having the courage to face life as it stands.

Acceptance that much of human society is founded on Perceptional Reality that leads to conflict.

Acceptance that there is much we cannot control in our lives, like our genetic inheritance and subconscious programs we have been taught as we grew to become adults.

Acceptance of our environment—social or political—in which we find ourselves, and that may be unhealthy and beyond our direct control.

Acceptance arises when we stop judging the perceptional world of conflict and our inherited past, which may not be congruent with health. We accept it in the knowledge that we cannot go back. Our past is our past. Now our focus shifts to the moment, and we use vital attention and balanced focus to continue our journey to a brighter future.

We not only accept, but we also forgive. We forgive others we feel may have done us wrong because we now understand it is simply an error of understanding that leads people astray. In the same vein we accept and forgive ourselves for the same errors we may have done, understanding they are the result of our own misconceptions about the nature of life.

We accept and forgive, not because it is right, not because we feel obliged to help others who we feel have done us wrong, but because it is the healthy thing to do. We simply realize that holding onto emotions of hurt and resentment does us harm, as it does harm to others. It creates internal emotional instability and conflict in ourselves that translates into physical imbalance, which then reflects out into the world. As the American pastor and writer, Harry Fosdick, expressed eloquently: "Hate. It is like burning down your own house to get rid of a rat."

The Flow of Vitality leads us into the experience of acceptance and forgiveness of ourselves and others. It creates an "eye in the storm" of life, a space in the way we see the world, which calms the emotional waves of conflict that so often blind us. We stop filling our moments with stress about a conflicted past. We stop being so anxious about an uncertain future. Instead, we start to fill this space with the experiences that Vitality brings. In so doing, we slowly shift our life onto a healthy path, and in earnest towards our health creation.

As we forgive, as we accept and embrace the 12 Principles of Health, we experience something deeper about the nature of life:

There is nothing to forgive.

Even in the world of perceptional conflict, life is always seeking equilibrium. Seeking to help us find our way back to the balance point that opens the door to our innate meaning and harmony—the place that makes us realize we are all connected.

Who we saw as enemies—our polar opposites—were really lighting up our own imbalanced perceptions of the world. Realizing this fundamental truth, we gain insight that life has always tried to show us a path towards health. This realization is the dawning of deep gratitude that heals the wounds in our hearts. Gratitude becomes the vehicle that changes our view of the world. Conflict is no longer who we are. Painful memories—as real as they may seem—are simply ghosts that hold only as much power over us as we give them.

We become free to stop fighting dualistic wars and reclaim responsibility for our lives. We stop becoming powerless victims. We don't risk becoming self-inflated heroes. We become more real. We do what has to be done to restore the balance and health of any situation.

American author and motivational speaker, Suze Orman, said it well when she stated: "When you are grateful—when you can see what you have—you unlock blessings to flow in your life."

This process is a transmutation of the way we see the world. It moves us from acceptance, through forgiveness, to gratitude, and creates and enables love to flow in our experience. Love becomes the experience that connects us to the world in a healthy manner. Love is the experience of Vitality flowing through our lives. It is a way of being that seeks to create health in the experience of life as a whole.

The world is no longer a scary, unfair, and imbalanced place. It is becoming balanced, meaningful, and engaging. Perceptional failures become learning cycles and experiences from which we grow more deeply as human beings. Perceptional enemies become people who help us deepen our commitment to the 12 Principles of Health, illuminating our own imbalanced perceptions. These help us grow towards health and embrace a richer, more fulfilling life.

As we step out of the matrix of Perceptional Reality and into the flow of Vitality, we begin to see that it is our own mind that has been creating our experience of Perceptional Reality. We can see through the illusion of the perceptional matrix that has kept us in a "prison" of conflicted experience for so long. We ourselves create the chains of this prison, and we ourselves hold the keys that set us free.

Our lives may be the same, but we are seeing life with new eyes. It's not what we are looking at that makes the difference, but *how* we see. Looking through the wisdom of our hearts, we begin to see the way life organizes itself in a healthy manner. We also notice something magical, something deeply mythical about the nature of life:

As we change the way we see, life changes with us.

Life understands us and is responding to our identity. It is striving to bring us what we are seeking. This vital experience helps us understand what the German theologian and philosopher, Master Eckhart, meant when he said that if he had only one prayer, it would be "Thank you".

Consciousness Fields: Resonance

*"We change the world not by what we say or do,
but as a consequence of what we have become."*

~ David R. Hawkins

In his insightful book, "Transcending the Fields of Consciousness", renowned psychiatrist and spiritual teacher, Dr. David Hawkins, discusses the various consciousness fields humans are capable of creating and experiencing. A core idea is that as a person moves closer to the consciousness of truth, their experience of life changes to become more in line with the underlying reality of life. These changes can be mapped on a field of experience, which he calls "fields of consciousness".

This map of experience closely correlates to the concept of Perceptional Reality, and the 12 Principles of Health. From my observations, consciousness fields that are below the level of truth and are perceptional in nature, erode health in our experience. They create a destructive matrix in our psychological and physical expression. The fields of consciousness that are in line with truth and express the 12 Principles of Health, are vital in nature. They hold true to the way life creates itself in a healthy manner.

*The journey to health in one's experience is a
journey to align who we are with the underlying
Vitality of life.*

Our health creation flows from the core of our being.

As Dr. Hawkins' quote states, we change our world—not by what we say or do—but by who we are. It is a matter of coming into resonance with the consciousness that flows health within us. Our thoughts and actions then flow from our state of being.

We have to let go of the states of being that are created from the perceptional world of duality. These states are like storm clouds that hide the real nature of Vitality, that hide our innate meaning, that throw us out of balance and destroy our harmony. These states create conflict and express illness in their experience.

We have to find the center of that storm. For in the eye of the perceptional storm resides a healthy state of being. These Vital Fields of being are like rays of sunlight that disperse the clouds of perception. They allow the light of Vitality to shine into our lives with increasing intensity. They illuminate health consciousness in our awareness. They unveil our innate meaning, help us stay balanced, and flow harmony into our lives. They are experiences that flow peace and love into our lives, and lead us to our health creation.

So let's take a short journey through the various "fields of consciousness" that we as humans experience, and explore how they relate to our health creation. As we remove the layers of distortion and build with the 12 Principles of Health, we see more clearly how our very own being creates our lives.

Vital Distortion:
Dualistic Embodiment

"When health is absent, wisdom cannot reveal itself, art cannot manifest, strength cannot fight, wealth becomes useless, and intelligence cannot be applied."

~ Herophilus

Although Vitality is always available to us, the mind has the ability to create experiential fields that are incongruent with health. These fields of reality are in essence energetic embodiments of distorted ideas, beliefs, and perceptions about life. These fields are incongruent with Vitality, simply because they do not reflect the principles upon which health stands, and they erode the Keys of Health in our experience.

These distorted perceptions are created when we embrace perceptional duality as our state of being. This identity then flows to become an expression in our minds, and is embodied as an emotional state.

Let's take a brief journey through the spectrum of these distorted experiential fields of consciousness that are so common in the human experience.

Perceptional Fields of Consciousness

Shame and Despair

This is perhaps the most distorted of the experiential fields that lack Vitality.

Within this perception, our sense of worth becomes absent in our experience. As a result, a person cannot see the meaning of their individual self, and the meaning of other people and objects. They are blinded by feelings of helplessness and hopelessness towards their situation, and are unable to see Vitality in their own experience.

The field creates a deep apathy and inability to take responsibility for one's own life. It is a lose-lose perception, which, when severe, is destructive to social bonds, and can even threaten physical survival due to a gravitation towards suicidal tendencies that it can create. Hope for a better future is perceived as being beyond one's ability to experience.

The end point of this field of experience is metaphorically similar to organ failure in its physical reflection. In organ failure, cells no longer carry out their required function, which means the organ cannot carry out its unique purpose. Because of the interdependent nature of the body this leads to detrimental effects upon the body as a whole, resulting in illness, and if severe enough, death.

Guilt and Hate

These are fields of experience that create dire imbalance and conflict in our relationships. They are created when meaning is gained from fighting a perceived evil from within, or from without.

When we perceive an enemy from within, we create **guilt**—a strong lose-win mentality, where one feels they are at fault in any given situation. This provokes thoughts of self-condemnation and punishment, which are detrimental to one's own well-being.

The perceptional distortion commonly creates its polar opposite, which expresses itself as **hate** of a perceived outside enemy. In this state, one feels the other is at fault and leads to emotional attack, and if severe, can lead to rage and killing as its physical expression. The expression of hate is a win-lose perception.

Often these experiences come together as a bipolar perception that switches from a lose-win to a win-lose mentality that creates the cycle of hate and guilt, and is embodied within this distorted energy field. The desire to harm one's self or another simply becomes two sides of the same coin. The result is relationship breakdown, emotional suffering, creation of social problems, and erosion of the Keys of Health.

In the physical reflection, this energy field of **guilt** can be likened to an autoimmune disease, where cells that were designed to protect the body turn on their own cells and destroy them, causing inflammation, damage, and illness.

Hate is akin to a viral or bacterial infection that enters the body with the sole purpose to destroy the host cells for its own gain. This leads to infection in the body that may lead to sepsis and death if severe enough.

Desire and Persistent Grief

These are common experiential fields that stem from the perceptional view that meaning and happiness is found in external sources. In this field of experience, meaning is no longer sourced from overcoming an enemy, but from attaining physical objects of desire. **Desire** becomes the driving force of our relationships.

Thus, because meaning is sourced from the world, the loss of a desired object, person or relationship leads to grief. We experience grief because we mistakenly believe we are losing that which is the source of our meaning and happiness.

Grief from loss can lead to despair if we are unable to obtain the object driving our meaning, such as the affection of another person. It may also lead to **anger** and **hate**, as the ego positions any person who it deems to have taken away its source of happiness as evil. A person may simply then choose another object to draw meaning from, and their experience may move back into **desire**.

A perceptional duality of win-lose and lose-win develops. We desire what we perceive will give us meaning and happiness—an experience of winning our happiness. We grieve when this perception is lost, feeling like we are losing, becoming angry at the perceived source of our loss, or to wallow in our despair. Only to again desire for another object we feel will give meaning or happiness.

This is embodied in the iconic "love-hate" relationships common to the human experience, which stems from great desire, leads to anguish, and often results in anger or despair when the relationship breaks down.

Metaphorically, in the physical reflection, this is expressed in any illness that derives from addiction to external substances, such as alcohol or drug dependency. Here, great desire for the object of perceived pleasure and meaning leads to grief when the person cannot get the substance of addiction. This in turn, leads to increasing desire.

Often the cycle of destruction deepens as desire and grief turn to anger and despair. Anger at anyone who keeps them from getting their substance of addiction and despair at the spiral of destruction the addiction is creating in their lives.

Addiction often leads to neglect of the essential needs of life, which are overridden by the need for the substance of addiction, thus leading to a slow derangement of social bonds, lifestyle, and physical illness.

Pride and Fear

These health-eroding perceptional fields are very common in our society and are hard to transcend. They are hard to see as perceptional because many believe fear to be useful and pride to be desirable.

Meaning in this polarity is sourced from an external position in the world. It stems from the belief or identity that the world is divided into winners and losers—those who have, and those who have-not. The meaning is to be a "winner" and attain objects of desire. If we are successful in attaining the objects of desire we experience a sense of **pride**.

Pride is an emotion of thinking one's self is better than others, which stems from a win-lose polarity. Yet pride is based on the external success of a person and thus is vulnerable to loss.

Pride is perceptional because its identity is created from an external comparative projection. Even within pride, its polar opposite, **fear**, is hiding—the fear of loss, of losing all that one has attained, fear of becoming a "loser". Social fear of losing status and one's accumulated possessions is sourcing an external meaning.

Because these two polarities are entangled, we can see how "pride comes before the fall", and "we attract what we fear". The greater the pride, the greater the fear of loss.

Fear becomes conscious when we find ourselves on the "losing" side of this polarity. We fear we are not enough, that we don't deserve to be winners. This may lead us to desire to become "winners", or to grieve over being a "loser". Sometimes we become angry at the "winners", feeling they have rigged the system to their ends, and start on a road to hate. This leads to conflict between these two polarities and creates imbalance in our society that leads to violence.

Other times we accept our lot as "losing" and fall into experiences of despair and shame at not being a "winner" in the game of life. This leads to dysfunction and tendencies towards self-harm. All of these pathways are perceptional and erode healthy expression in our experience.

The perceptional fields of pride and fear lead to a desperate desire to have more—at the expense of relationship balance. As balance and harmony are eroded, health suffers. People with pride cling to their status, while those who lack pride and are driven by fear rise up to revolt or suffer anxiety that drives them towards despair and shame of being "losers" in the game of life.

Pride is perhaps the hardest perceptional field of experience to leave behind because it feels good. It feels as if we have finally made it. Realizing that we have only found another mirage in the desert is difficult to accept.

This perceptional growth of having more—to be a "winner"—lacks vision of the interdependent nature of life.

The win-lose mentality of pride and the lose-win mentality of fear is akin to cancer cells that grow and divide without heeding the needs of other cells in the body—driven by pride and the subconscious fear of loss. They deplete the energy of other cell systems through lack of resources. This leads to inflammation and destruction of cells as the body defends itself from erosion. If successful, cancer cells cause damage to the body as a whole, which ends up also causing the demise of the cancer cells because they are also part of the body's system.

Having explored the emotional, perceptional experiences that create distortion in our relationships and erode health in our experience, let us now embark on a journey through the center of the polar opposites. Here, where the flow of life is deepest, we begin to awaken to a new way of experiencing the world.

We begin to see life as it stands, rather than as we perceive it.

Let's look at the consciousness fields of experience that flow from Vitality and create our lives in a healthy manner.

Consciousness Fields of Health:
Vitality Experience

"When love awakens in your life, in the night of your heart,
it is like the dawn breaking within you.
When before there was anonymity, now there is intimacy;
Where before there was fear, now there is courage;
Where before in your life there was awkwardness,
now there is a rhythm of grace and gracefulness;
Where before you used to be jagged,
now you are elegant and in rhythm with your self.
When love awakens in your life, it is like a rebirth, a new beginning."

~ John O'Donohue

Let us now move deeper toward the vital dimension. Let us add color to the bipolar black-and-white world of perception. Let us see how health principles are expressed in our emotional experience to unveil Vitality in our own being.

As we move through the fields of experience that embody the 12 Principles of Health, we begin to notice that life begins to embrace Vitality in its experience—health and life begin to merge. In the end, we are simply discovering who it is we really are. On our journey to the center of our own being, we begin to embody different ways of seeing the world. We begin to embody a sense of responsibility, acceptance, creativity, relationship awareness, and ultimately spiritual insight. On our journey to health, we realize life is a wonderful expression of love. That the peace humanity has been seeking for so long has been here all along, just waiting for us to open our eyes and see its reality flowing within us.

Courage

Courage is reflected in the principle of **awareness**. It is the commitment to look at life as it stands. It is the realization that one must take responsibility for one's own life and that meaning arises from within. It is embodied in the rejection of the dualistic, Perceptional Reality, and solidified by finding one's internal **security** in making a commitment to embrace life, in principle, in one's own experience.

Courage occurs as an experience when the first two principles of Awareness and Security are embodied into one's reality. The energy field created is one of strength and stability, and forms a platform on which to build our experience of health.

In the body this is reflected in the ability of cells to become health-focused, and thus to do what needs to be done to maintain a healthy balance within the context of their own reality. It is expressed by the creation of cell membranes. Cell membranes are a semi-permeable boundary that is key to the health of every cell. It embraces nutrients and rejects toxins, and creates a stable internal core from which a cell can operate. It is the security which sets the tone for healthy expression.

Neutrality

Neutrality is a field of consciousness that is created when a person becomes "okay" with life as it stands. That is, when we cease to judge the world of perception.

Like courage, this field is founded on the realization that meaning derives from an internal source, and thus precedes external circumstances. This field is embodied when the principle of internal **power** is combined with that of **security**. This comes about when a person stops grasping at objects of desire, and stops emotionally fighting objects of threat, and begins to find emotional **equanimity** in their outlook.

Equanimity, allows a person not to react to perceptional attack, since they no longer take such attacks personally, realizing they arise from a perceptional construct that no longer serves them. This outlook becomes the foundation of a stable emotional core from which clarity of any given situation can be sought. This clarity gives us the ability to respond to situations in a considerate manner.

In the physical body, this is metaphorically reflected in a cell's capacity to respond to its environment in a manner that is focused on preserving stable integrity of its function, no matter what stimulus is being presented. Like a river that flows around obstacles, rather than fighting them, neutrality allows an individual to choose the path most congruent with a healthy outcome. Here, people realize that every circumstance can be seen in many different ways, yet in the end, choosing a healthy path is more important than being right. As such, their focus begins to be less on reacting to perceptional positions, and more on context—making sure one is seeing and interacting with life in a healthy manner.

Mother Teresa once said that if you judge people, you have not time to love them. This sentiment becomes self-evident when we embody a sense of neutrality in our lives.

Willingness

Willingness is an energy field that embraces the principle of **balancing one's own hemispheres**. It stands on the shoulders of courage and neutrality. Here, the ability to balance the creative right hemisphere with the logical left hemisphere of our minds enables one to become the creative leader of one's own life, while using reason to plan and execute around the leadership decisions. This creates an inner drive to engage life, and leads to the ability to self-govern, and thus is a foundation for one's independence. People become reliable team players. Willingness moves people to have an intention for an engaged and healthy contribution to life.

In the physical reflection, this is akin to cells balancing their ability to create the right proteins and organic materials that help them function effectively in their environment, with the genetic precision of expression that drives this process. In physical cellular reality, this ability reflects the foundation for the autonomy and independence of a healthy living cell in its expression.

Acceptance

Acceptance is the consciousness state that we embody when we become aware that we are the source and the creators of our experience, and that creation flows from inside to out. We accept the world as it is, knowing that fighting perceptional battles only erodes our own health. We begin to build our lives from within—both in our actions and in the way we create our emotional well-being. We begin to create ourselves in a healthy manner.

This field of experience is embodied through the principle of **emotional alchemy**, and the realization of **our own uniqueness**. Realizing that meaning is found within, we begin to create our own happiness by establishing confidence and well-being from an internal pathway as **emotional alchemy** is embraced in one's experience.

Instead of fighting the world, we draw on our internal resources to awaken our **unique** purpose, which we then express in the world. When acceptance is reached as an energetic state of being, one embodies the masculine principles that create our **independence**. The experience is one of an explorer who has the resources and confidence to go out into the world and to interact with our environment in an engaging manner. It sets the foundations for productive and creative contribution in our lives and in our society.

In the body this is metaphorically reflected as an independent, healthy cell that has specialized to be a part of an organ system. This system then contributes in a unique way to serve the body as a whole. Be it a heart cell that helps to pump blood to supply nutrients, a kidney cell that filters toxins, or a skin cell that protects the internal environment. Acceptance of who we are and engagement to live life as it stands enables a cell to express its independence in a healthy manner.

Reason

Reason is the consciousness state that begins to reach out and explore the reality of interaction from a position of independence. Having found internal meaning and balance, reason looks out to expand this within the context of relationships. This is done through the mechanism of understanding how life functions. Reason strives to look at life as it stands, understand how it functions, and at its most noble, embody the **Triple-Win principle**—seeking to find ways to interact that are beneficial for all involved.

Reason is the field of awareness from which science arose. Western medicine, psychology, law, and philosophy were all created from the field of reason, in the striving to correct imbalance in human social interaction, and in our own bodies and mind so that social order, and physical health may prevail once more. Reason has done much to alleviate the suffering of humanity.

Democracy was also founded in this field of consciousness. This is why democracy, at its most noble, seeks to create systems to benefit the most people in society at any given time.

Within the body, reason is metaphorically akin to the central nervous system, whose function it is to collect data on the needs of all body parts, and create and distribute resources in a way that meets the needs of all. When we embody Triple-Win as a lifestyle, we set the stage for health to prevail in one's experience.

The field of reason, however, is limited by the linear system on which it is founded. Something deeper must arise for reason to prevail in its quest to find a healthy solution to the complexity of interaction of living things. Here, we find ourselves at another evolutionary leap of consciousness.

Love

Love is created when one embodies the principle of **synergy** into one's experience. Love is the greatest stepping stone that opens up the flow of Vitality. This non-local field sees how living things unify, and begins to flow harmony into our relationships. The walls of separation begin to tumble down, and the balance of **Triple-Win** is created along a harmonious middle path that is synergistic to both sides. It is the mythical union where two become one. Our internal meaning and purpose begin to merge with the meaning and purpose of others, creating deeper connections, and forming harmonious relationships that are held in place by the field of Vitality that connects and unifies living things.

> *Your health creation starts to become an experience*
> *that flows out into your life when love is present as*
> *a context of seeing and being in the world.*

The experience of joy and deeper meaning become natural states that do not disappear when life does not go to plan, and troubles arise. One begins to experience that life seeks to support one's visions and dreams because they, themselves, are life-supporting.

The experience of love is felt and orchestrated by the heart. Unlike reason, which sees the pieces and seeks to put them together in ways that create a whole, love sees the whole. Love is able to see the value and meaning of every piece.

The integration of the heart with the mind is the dawning of love.

The whole becomes more than the sum of its parts, and the expression of spontaneous health creation becomes a possibility.

In the physical, this energetic field seeks to create harmony through synergistic pathways, and is expressed in our autonomic nervous systems and endocrine systems that operate the body under the level of conscious awareness. They are aware of the needs of the body as a whole and seek to organize resources and create the body in a unified manner, which benefits all healthy cells. Their actions are spontaneous and in keeping with the intelligence field of Vitality that orchestrates their action.

Unconditional Love

Unconditional love evolves as an experience when the principle of embracing the **Cycles of Life** becomes integrated in one's experience. In this state, the connection to Vitality deepens and stabilizes as one sees that everything in life is connected and flows in natural rhythms and cycles. We become accepting of endings, knowing they are simply doorways to new beginnings. This is experienced as a state of grace—a flow of life that moves us increasingly into experiences of harmony in the way we structure our lives. We find ourselves flowing through life in a way that connects us to others in meaningful ways and brings joy into our lives

Embracing the **order** that the 12 Principles of Health create, allows for ever-increasing experiences of **freedom** within our lives, as doors open up from where there had only been walls. Life becomes an increasingly mysterious experience. Serendipity and seemingly miraculous coincidences become a common experience.

These miracles are now simply connections manifesting from an unseen connection to all life—one that we are now conscious of. They flow into our experience because we are aligning our lives with Vitality and becoming keenly aware of the underlying spiritual nature of life, and the innate interconnection of all living systems. Vitality is no longer an idea, but something truly flowing within our experience.

Physically, this reflects the cell cycle that enables growth and maturation of the body and connects cells in an interdependent manner. It is the presence of the circulation driven by the heart to ensure distribution of nutrients and oxygen to all cells in the body. These forces unite the body, creating it in cycles of renewal and rejuvenation, and embrace the impermanence of life as a natural expression of a healthy physical existence.

As cells naturally begin to align with the energetic Vitality in their physical expression, health creation starts to filter in as a real experience, and we experience ourselves belonging to life as a whole. There is a natural experience of joy and freedom that results from a healthy life.

Peace

Peace as an experience is the result of the consciousness state that has embraced Vitality completely. It is created from all of the 12 Principles of Health, as they begin to **translate into the physical world**. When Vitality is experienced as a flow in our lives it becomes clear that it arises from a place that cannot be lost—it arises from life itself. We are simply a part of this greater whole.

The polarity of life and death becomes illuminated as an illusion. It may be that our bodies and minds follow the cycles of birth and death that belong to the cycles of life on this planet, but our lives flow from a deeper reality held within a vital field of life that cannot be destroyed. When we experience this "sanctum" of our being directly, there is a sense of peace and calm that is created in our experience of life.

We begin to see that everything in our lives serve our deeper purpose, and that we belong to a life that is intimate, holds within it great meaning, connection, and love. We begin to feel gratitude and a sense of coming home to where we belong—finding our innate selves within the experience of life.

We become free to **make a stand** for the health of all living systems, to embrace our health creation, and to flow our meaning and creativity into the world with courage.

When we see our reality flows from a place that cannot be distorted by Perceptional Reality—that indeed our essence belongs to this place that cannot be destroyed nor corrupted—we become free to live our lives in a peaceful manner.

SECTION 4
MANIFESTATIONS OF VITALITY IN THE PHYSICAL WORLD

Expressions of Vitality

"People say that all we're seeking is a meaning for life. I don't think that's what we're really seeking. I think that what we're really seeking is an experience of being alive, so that our life experiences on the purely physical plane will have resonance with our own innermost being and reality, so that we actually feel the rapture of being alive."

~ Joseph Campbell

When perceptions are frozen within a dualistic matrix, a black-and-white reality is created in the way we see the world that leads to distortion, imbalance, and loss of health. This perception creates a conflicted experience in our lives, where emotions of pride, fear, apathy, desire, and anger begin to dominate our lives. In this state we are unable to create a life of meaning. We keep losing our balance, and conflicts in our lives make it difficult to reach our goals. We lose our expression of health within the matrix of our perceptional experience.

Our experience of Vitality is like adding color to the perceptional world; suddenly polarity is transformed into colorful expressions that can be put together in a vast array of ways. The "color" sparks creativity and forges harmony upon which healthy expression is founded.

Vitality weaves a dynamic dimension to the intelligence of health. As health principles are energetically embodied into physical expressions in time and space, they create an animated reality in our experience. We find our courage, and feel motivated to contribute to the world. We engage with our lives with creative reason, and are lifted to reach our goals. We are moved to live our lives in a healthy manner. The result is an artistic expression, infused with meaning and balance; a harmonious expression that captures within it the experience of joy and love. It brings peace to our souls.

Vitality flows from the heart and creates in our experience the rapture of being alive.

Let us now explore a few key areas in life where we can "tune in" to Vitality as it operates around us. These examples capture vitality because they flow the intelligence of health as an expression into the physical world.

The Symphony of Life:
The Vitality of Sound

"Harmony sinks deep into the recesses of the soul and takes its strongest hold there, bringing grace also to the body, and the mind as well. Music is a moral law. It gives a soul to the universe, wings to the mind, flight to the imagination, a charm to sadness, and life to everything. It is the essence of order ..."

~ Plato (429-347)

If health was a great symphony, then the instruments would be the individuals of life. Each instrument is **independent** in scope, yet they have to play in an **interdependent** manner within the orchestra to create a musical piece that is greater than the sum of each individual part.

In other words, they have to adapt the 12 Principles of Health to create meaning, balance, and harmony in their expression. Together they can create a musical piece that carries within it the vital energy that evokes inspiration and joy within the listener.

Let us have a closer look at how the symphony is founded on the principles that govern health.

Looking at a Symphony Through Vital Attention

The instruments are created with an **awareness** of their innate **meaning**, and how they are to belong to the orchestra in a vital manner. This understanding sets the platform for healthy musical expression. It gives them the innate potential that will bring the symphony to life.

They are required to be of unique anatomical shape and size to be able to play their unique sound that is in harmony with the other instruments. This physical definition is their **security** and **power**. It is founded in the "courage" of self expression—a sense of being "okay" with who they are—knowing that their unique identity flows from the innate knowledge of their Vitality.

A **balance of creativity and reason** must go into their creation and musical expression. The **creativity** is in the choosing of their design, shape, and material from which they are built. The **reason** is in the actions that must be taken to create them from the raw materials of life. This action is the willingness to engage in life, inspired by the creative impulse that flows from Vitality within.

When an instrument is complete, tuned, and played with **confidence**, it gives off a sound that carries within it a sense of **well-being**. This expression of sound creates a sense of happiness felt when listening to a well-played instrument—a form of **emotional alchemy** that is created from the instrument's innate nature.

There are many **unique** instruments that make up a great symphony. Some, like the woodwinds, play high and sweet tunes, and others, like the brass, are booming and strong. The strings are emotional in their expression, while the percussion creates a sense of rhythm. In a great symphony, all of them are as valuable as each other. A created instrument, is an **independent** individual within the world of the orchestra. Each one brings their unique qualities, an acceptance of who they are, and a willingness to express their uniqueness to contribute to something greater. Only by playing together in a **balanced** and considerate manner can they create the **harmony** of a moving piece of music.

It is the way they relate that is the making or breaking of a great piece of music. They must play in a way that complements each other; to reason themselves to consociate in ways where sounds blend and add to each other's values; to strike a **balance** of **volume** as they connect to each other and to the audience who is listening.

This balance and complement of sound with other instruments and the audience enables the **Triple-Win principle** to prevail that allows the orchestra to play in a manner that avoids conflict of sound and is uplifting for all involved.

When instruments play in harmony, when they come into a rhythm that appeals to the ear, when their sounds blend to create a single piece of music, there is a **synergistic** experience taking place. A vibrant unified piece of music is being held together by vital expression that enables individual instruments to belong to something greater than one's own individual expression. This synergy of sound carries within it the magical experience that opens up feelings of love and joy to those who listen to true masterpieces of music.

Continuing this analogy, a symphony can be as **free** in its composition as the composer's imagination allows. Yet within this freedom it must adhere to a set of **ordered musical principles** for it to be deemed a beautiful piece of music. By embracing the order of health, the composer is given freedom to express their own musical creation. It is the meaning, the balance, and the harmony that is creating the joyful expression within the piece of music that sets the music free in its creativity. The Vitality of sound becomes the portal for freedom of the musical expression.

As the music weaves its harmony, it follows cycles of repetition which reflect the **Cycles of Life**. The music begins, evolves, and grows to maturity through cycles as more instruments join to add depth to the piece. Yet songs do not play forever. They reach a climax, and move on to fade into a gratifying ending, signaling the closure of the cycle. There, in the silence, the audience waits for the next song to begin. Even within the silence the gentle presence of Vitality creates a space of potentiality—a peaceful knowing that music can be set free once more to express itself in a vital manner.

It is the composer who has **made a stand** to ensure vital expression of the symphony by eliminating sounds that are incongruent with harmony, and choosing only combinations that are balanced and meaningful in their expression.

The composer is the heart that is listening to the wisdom of Vitality that is flowing within life and all around us.

Not all pieces of music created are masterpieces, yet when "mistakes" are made, and harmony and balance are disrupted, it becomes clear to the listener.

However, these "errors" are simply learning cycles. Through such "errors" the composer, conductor, and players learn how to create on a more vital level. They **make a stand** to focus their attention on the creation of a great symphony rather than the judgement of errors. This allows them to grow and become great artists.

It is the conductor who **translates all these principles into physical reality** by directing the instruments to flow the harmony of the piece in space and time. The conductor is the mind that is translating the wisdom of the heart into physical expression. The instruments are the physical body expressing the creation.

The heart feels the Vitality of the music, creating it, for the mind to flow it into the orchestra in the moment, sparking the creation of the piece of music that moves us from within.

Although this is a metaphor for health, music is a reflection of the nature of Vitality. As Plato noted many years ago: "Music is a moral law ... that brings grace to the body and the mind".

When we listen to great pieces such as Pachelbel's canon in D, Mozart's Eine Kleine Nachtmusik (The Night

Music), and Vivaldi's Four Seasons, we are moved by their power. They resonate with our hearts, and bring with them an experience of joy, which touches the innate wisdom of love.

Such compositions have the ability to put us into into a state of consciousness from which they are created. We relax, our feelings deepen, and our mind finds peace within the context of the musical expression. The autonomic nervous systems gravitates to balance. For a few minutes, a portal into the dimension of Vitality swings open, and we are free to bask in its light. It is a river of sound leading our consciousness back to the center, where health resides. It's easy to feel a sense of gratitude and connection when one is in this space of being.

The Vitality of Movement:
The Dance of Life

"Dance is the hidden language of the soul."

~ Martha Graham

Life is movement. For life to be healthy, it requires its movement to be infused with vital intelligence. When this happens, movement takes on an artistic flair, and health is made manifest in physical form. To watch a dancer who has mastered their art is to watch Vitality animated.

At its most vital, dancing is an animated expression of health within space and time.

Experiencing Dancing Through Vital Attention

The dance begins in stillness, silence, yet the **awareness** of the expression about to unfold is already there. The field of Vitality is already present within us, waiting for it to be expressed in a physical manner.

The dance is created on a platform of cultivated poise and balance that the dancer has embodied in their expression. These create the **security** that the dancer uses to form a foundation for vital movement—the courage of self-expression.

As the music starts the dancer "tunes in" to the moment of creation from which the dance unfolds. The focus is not in the past, nor is it in the future. It is collapsed into the creative moment. This equanimity of focus gives the dancer their **power** for vital expression. It holds within it the knowing that it is "okay" to be seen as we are.

As the music plays, the dancer's mind captures vital awareness within the rhythms and the harmonies of the song. This inspires creativity of movement; a willingness for self-expression.

The creativity is held in balance by the mind of reason that enacts the movements in space and time. This **balancing of the creative and logical aspects of the mind** allows for the dance to unfold in a creative and effective manner.

The joy of the dance wells up as an innate expression. The **emotional alchemy** of embracing confidence in the steps of the dance with the well-being of creative expression, creates a sense of joy one feels when seeing a great dancer, or when we dance in a vital manner. It creates happiness from within, that is expressed in the form of dancing.

In full flight we create the dance in the moment. Each step is our own. No two people on the dance floor dance exactly the same, yet all dance with a passion of their own **uniqueness** expressed within the rhythms and harmonies of the song. There is no "right" or "wrong" dance. There is only dancing that reaches ever deeper and connects us to our innate nature. We find acceptance of who we are as a dancer and a knowledge that we belong on the stage of life.

Yet as we dance, we are not dancing alone. Dance is often created with a partner you have chosen to engage with. There are also many others occupying the dance floor, sharing the space of expression. Your partner's steps are unique, as are those of everyone else. Yet you know you are dancing for a common purpose: to embrace the beauty of life and enhance joy in each other's experience. This joy can be felt by others. This reasoning of dancing that brings benefit to everyone embodies the **Triple-Win** principle and creates a sense of community and interdependent connection.

As we embrace the dance with our being, we enter an experience where we are no longer just dancing as a single individual. The space and time between you and your partner collapses, and the experience of **synergy** with your partner, and others on the dance floor is created. A unification takes place. A connection on an emotional and visceral level that pulses love and a sense of belonging into the experience. We feel connected to each other, to the community. We belong to something greater than our own individual expression. We feel the flow of Vitality connect us to the dance. There is a mysterious communion taking place, flowing love into our hearts and out into the world, and making dancing a heartfelt experience.

The dance floor is an open stage. You are free to express in any way you please, as long as the harmony of the dance is maintained. In that space, one can see the **freedom of expression** flowing within the order of Vitality that has created it.

The feeling of freedom is expansive. The dance builds in ever more complex moves created by your imagination—and the imaginations of everyone on the dance floor—and held in harmony by the Vitality of the music that animates your dance. You are going nowhere, but then again now-here is all you ever needed to realize the freedom that resides within the depths of your own heart. There is joy flowing within that freedom.

However, the song must end, as all songs do.

The stage returns to silence, the communion between you and your partner ends as you exit the dance floor. Yet your heart is inspired, your mind is enthused. You know this is simply another **cycle of life**. The next song will come, a new dance will arise. The joy of dancing will continue.

There's a sense of unconditional love in knowing that the Vitality that drives joyful expression does not disappear, but rather stays within us, anticipating the flow into a new expression, marking the new cycle of a new dance in life.

Even as you leave the dance club into the darkness of a solemn street at the end of a night of dancing, you are still dancing inside. The connection to life, forged by the experience of Vitality lingers on in your awareness. There is the opportunity to translate the "dance" **into your life** now. You're **Making a Stand** to make a dance out of your life. For, in a way, life was always meant to be a dance. There is gratitude in that understanding.

Life was not meant to be a conflicted struggle. Rather, it is a process of health creation that springs from a river of vital energy that flows love into our lives, and brings peace to our hearts and minds.

As Martha Graham noted, "Dance is the hidden language of the soul".

Nature: The Wilderness Within

"Nature always wears the colors of the spirit."

~ Ralph Waldo Emerson

The term nature refers to the sum of all living systems existing together in an interdependent manner, which we term an ecosystem.

Although humans have separated themselves from the natural environment in many ways, our health is interwoven with nature. Life is a web of interconnected living things. On the physical level, this is reflected in our need for clean water that we obtain from rivers and lakes, nutritious food that we grow from fertile soil, and the clean air and oxygen created by the forests and grasslands of the world.

On an energetic level, nature, like all living systems, shares a common identity. Its expressions are founded on principles that allow it to create itself in a healthy manner. One can feel the presence of this vital expression when spending time in a rich, natural environment.

So, let's take a stroll into the mountains and explore the Vitality of nature.

Looking at Nature Through Vital Attention

It is sunrise over the snow-capped mountains. Watching the peaks burn with a golden hue as they are illuminated by the rising sun creates a stillness within. Our **awareness** is transported into a presence of a grounded knowing.

The mountains have been there for millions of years. Their rocky foundations speak of courage, patience, fortitude, and a deep sense of **independence**. **Security** and **power** is their expression. The mountains know who they are and how they belong. They do not require anything outside of themselves to affirm their mighty reality. Nor do they judge. In their neutrality, they are simply okay with the way the world revolves around them.

Sunrise passes and the day springs to life in earnest.

Walking down the mountain path you begin to notice that even as the mountains embrace a core stability of independent existence, their surface is covered in life, full of creative and interactive intensity—an array of plants, trees, animals, and insects. A symphony of living things weave a web of creative complexity that is hard to comprehend with the logical mind, yet the heart can feel and appreciate with a silent understanding.

As one walks on, enjoying this symphony of life, one cannot help but smile at the wonder of nature. There is a deep sense of **confidence** that wells up from the natural environment—confidence to engage and live life fully.

There is also a sense of **well-being**—a knowing of one's place in the natural world. It is a belonging that evokes happiness within our hearts and speaks to the emotional alchemy present in nature.

Looking closer, every living thing—no matter how **unique** its expression—balances **creativity** and **reason**. Creativity in the way it expresses its own steps within the greater dance of the mountain life. Carried out with reason to ensure its needs are met and secured. It expresses a willingness to contribute to the ecosystem of the mountain life.

We walk towards a tall and mighty waterfall with a sense of purpose and clarity of self-identity. The waters sweep over the rocky walls far above and fall down into a fresh pool of water, to then turn into a flowing stream. One can feel the powerful force of falling water as it roars downwards. The waters have been shaping this land for thousands of years. A timeless presence is felt, for a human lifetime is a mere moment in the life of the waterfall.

As much as the water shapes the land, it also yields. The flow of the stream, fed by the falling water, does not fight the many obstacles in its way. It seeks out pathways that benefit its purpose to flow onwards towards the ocean. It chooses ways to flow around obstacles—a path of least resistance. The stream provides nourishment to all the plants and animals that live around it. It reminds us that nature seeks pathways that benefit itself and others, capturing the **Triple-Win** principle in its natural expression.

We too are flowing down the River of Life towards our destination. Like the water, we can choose to seek paths that are mutually beneficial to us, others, and the environment. We remain in the flow of life and embody it, energizing us from within and enabling us to flow towards our health creation.

We leave the waterfall and enter the forest at the feet of the mighty mountains. We feel the unity of the living ecosystems of which we are now a part. Even though the forest is made of many different and unique individual living things, they co-exist, in an interdependent manner. This **synergy** of spirit sparks feelings of love towards the natural world, towards life itself.

Walking along the path we see a young sapling growing from the rich soil in the undergrowth. Its energy is vibrant as it reaches for the sky. Not long ago it was but a seed. Its journey has just begun.

A large tree stands next to it. It has experienced many seasons of growth and evolution.

An old dying tree lies on the forest floor nearby. Its body is returning back to the earth, making room for new saplings to sprout. Its decomposing body provides shelter for animals and lays the foundation for a fertile soil that will support the next generation of trees.

The **Circle of Life**, embodied in the life cycle of the tree, inspires us to become a little wiser in the way we relate to the time we have and the seasons of our own lives. They speak of inspiration and new beginnings, growth and patience, acceptance of endings, and the natural rhythms of life. They evoke feelings of unconditional love towards our own lives—a deeper sense of belonging.

There is a **freedom** in nature—a freedom that puts the "wild" into wilderness. Yet as much as freedom of expression is granted, the natural world still adheres to the **order of health**. It ensures it is able to build itself in a sustainable manner that is supportive of all life forms within every ecosystem.

The individual life forms are **Making a Stand** to live, grow, and thrive—to translate their expression into their lives. They co-exist with each other. For only together can the ecosystem continue in a healthy manner. There is an acceptance and an embracing of life as it stands. There is a love pulsing through every living system. It is an uncanny **peace** felt in one's heart—a peace within the eye of the storm of life. It is a gratitude for life itself.

Leaving the forest and entering a clearing, it is nearly sunset. The songs of the frogs and insects pulsate through the warm air, filled with vibrant life. Walking to a pond in the middle of the clearing, orange hues on its waters reflect the sun as it slips behind the mountainous horizon.

A mountain hut is just ahead. A fire is waiting: food and shelter. Our experiences are not simply memories, **they become us**. The fire lit within one's heart keeps the soul warm.

As the nineteenth Century American poet, Ralph Waldo Emerson, noted: "Nature always wears the colors of the spirit". Within nature resides the magic of Vitality, and health is its expression.

Meditative Silence:
Communion with Our Vital Nature

*A Buddhist monk was asked: "What have you
gained from meditation?"
"Nothing," he replied. "However, let me tell you
what I have lost: anger, anxiety, depression,
insecurity, fear of old age, and death."*

~ Unknown

The discipline of meditation is perhaps the most simple and subtle expression of Vitality. The aim is simply to connect in one's awareness to the flow of Vitality present within us.

As we become still on the inside, the world of perceptions arise within us. As we stay in this state of awareness, the perceptions begin to fall away, and the reality of Vitality begins to shine through the perceptional paradigms of our own minds.

When meditation is practiced, and one's experience becomes aligned with Vitality, there is a transformation in the way we relate to life. We begin to connect to life directly. We begin to experience the intelligence of health as it flows from within.

This experience leads to a transformation that is life-changing, by gravitating your life towards a healthy expression. Feelings of compassion, love, and a deep sense of inner peace are common.

Conflicts decrease in frequency and intensity as one becomes increasingly secure in their independence, and creative in the way they form synergistic relationships. The experience can seem somewhat miraculous to people who are used to internal and external conflict being a normal state of experience. It seems miraculous because you begin to experience a process of inner creation that does not depend on external circumstances.

It is not the world that is driving the change. All that is changing is one's awareness of the reality that already exists within. This reality, of something greater than "I", governs our health, and shines through our inner stillness. Because of the interconnection of life, as you change your inner identity, the world changes with you. Your health creation has a ripple effect on your life, that evolves in a natural and synergistic manner.

Meditation is the art of "tuning in" to the field of Vitality. It is a reality of experience that cuts through the dualistic perceptions that erode health. Meditation does not create health—it unearths it in our experience. It is already within us. When we become aware of its presence, it affects our thoughts, feelings, and actions. It becomes the foundation stone to your health creation.

The great artist Michelangelo was once asked about one of his famous pieces of art:

"How did you create the statue of David?"

To which he replied:

"I did not create him, I simply set him free."

He did so, by simply chipping at a block of stone until David remained.

So too it is with meditative silence. It chips away at all that is unhealthy, until only love and peace remain. The monk's wise words reflect this truth: "I gained nothing," he said, knowing that Vitality has always been within him. "But let me tell you what I have lost …"

Vitality: Conclusion

"Life is art ... paint your dreams."

~ Unknown

Vitality is the intelligent energy that animates health in living organisms. Its principles are universal, yet its influence on our lives is deeply personal.

Humans are a very unique animal species. Our uniqueness stems from our ability to imagine and dream, to create our own identity, and to change and adapt quickly. We have the capacity for introspection.

Because of this ability of self-awareness and self-determination, we experience Vitality as a creative force, which has the power to build our dreams in a healthy manner. We experience it as an intelligent relationship to life. It is a guide that steers our hearts and minds in ways that set us on a mythological journey to create a meaningful life that fulfills our dreams.

The more we embrace its reality, the more we are able to create health in our own lives. Because its presence decreases conflict, our health creation becomes effective and efficient. Collectively, we become able to create healthy social systems and a healthy society. Globally, Vitality can flow our relationships to the natural world in ways that ensure the health of the planet.

"Life is art ... paint your dreams," is a statement that reflects our relationship with the intelligence that governs health in our experience. Vitality is expressed as art. It enables us to paint our dreams on the canvas of life. Yet it creates our lives in a manner that also builds the dreams of others, and supports the dreaming of the natural environment to which we belong.

Vitality is the field of intelligence that animates health in living organisms. It flows from our souls, from the "Sanctum" that resides deep within. Let us explore this Sanctum, which is so hard to remember, and yet when experienced, impossible to forget.

Summary of Vitality:

1. Vitality is the term I use to capture the flow of health intelligence expressed in the physical manner, through the various energies that animate a healthy living organism.

2. Vitality is felt as an expression in the heart. It is the integration of our hearts with our minds, that enables us to connect with Vitality, that drives our own health creation.

3. Vitality is always present where life exists. It is what allows life to create itself, to grow, to evolve, to reproduce, and to integrate within the ecosystems we see on the planet.

4. The experience of Vitality enables spontaneous health creation to act in our lives, on the level of our bodies, our minds, our social expression, and the world at large.

5. As vitality grows in our expression, it transforms our experiences from conflicted, perceptional realities, founded on fear, despair, desire, and pride, towards finding courage and acceptance of our world. We find a willingness to contribute and reason in the way we interact. Vitality lifts us into the experiences of love and joy that allow creativity of expression and inspiration. It has the power to bring us the experience of peace—even within a conflicted world.

6. We can find Vitalities echo in the artistic expression of music and dance. We connect to its flow when we immerse ourselves in the natural world. Yet, we do not need to do

anything to realize its reality, for it is already present within us. We can go within and feel it in the silence of our being as we listen to the rhythms of our hearts.

7. Within the order of Vitality resides the keys to our freedom—freedom to express our uniqueness, freedom to build loving relationships, freedom to achieve our goals and dreams, and the freedom to ensure this planet is not destroyed by the actions of Perceptional Reality. Vitality is the foundation of life. Deep within us, there is a place from which Vitality flows. It is the Sanctum of our being.

Chapter 8

Sanctum

Integration of the Human Soul

*"Even after all this time the sun never says to the
earth, 'you owe me'.
Look what happens to a love like that.
It lights the whole sky ..."*

~ Hafiz

This last chapter looks at what can be called the **Spiritual Dimension** of health. I call it the **Sanctum** of our being.

The Sanctum can be thought of as a mythological place that resides within human consciousness. It holds the keys to our health creation. It is the soul of the human experience from which Vitality flows.

The Sanctum resides as a core identity at the heart of life. It resides unseen, outside of the boundaries of space and time. The flow of its identity is always from in to out, and as such, this mysterious place is never disturbed by the perceptional fluctuations of the psychological or physical realities.

In the world of thought and matter, the apparent chain of cause and effect makes reality susceptible to perceptional disturbance. These disturbances can erode the Keys of Health, and result in illness—in all of its physical, psychological, and social expressions.

Yet within the Sanctum, cause and effect disappears. Life arises as a creation, as a gift. Its meaning, balance, and harmony is never disturbed. From such a place, the body and mind are created in a healthy manner because its intelligence flows outwards as the field of Vitality that guides creative potential. It is a seamless connection of organic matter, energy, and the intelligence that guides our health creation.

The Unmoved Mover

The Sanctum never seeks anything, for it holds within it, the keys to life. It is already whole, holding all the pieces of creation in its reality. It is still, unmoved by the fluctuations of the perceptional world. It is at peace. Yet, it is connected to everything, flowing its presence into the world through the expression of Vitality.

This metaphysical place can be likened to the Sun. It lies at the center, forever shining outwards, and providing the energy required for all of life, yet never requiring anything in return. Poetically, we can feel the magnitude of such an experience. The famous Persian poet, Hafiz, eludes to this place that lies at the heart of the human experience when he wrote: "Look at what happens to a love like that. It lights the whole sky."

The Health Spectrum

Another analogy is "light" as a metaphorical representation of the Sanctum. The Sanctum is white light, and life is the spectrum of colors, each with their own unique expression. When the spectrum of colors pass through a prism they unite to form white light. Similarly, the Sanctum holds within its reality all the expressions of life.

Our health consciousness becomes a prism that bends all the elements of life in such a manner that creates a unified reality. This is the awareness of the Sanctum in our experience. In the Sanctum, all life is unified and in a state of peace.

However, the process is actually an inversion of light through the prism: it is the Sanctum passing through the prism of our consciousness to create the health spectrum, which is held in unified diversity by the field of Vitality. The essence of reality is a unified one.

The appearance of separation is an illusion. The absence of health is simply a disconnection from Vitality that flows from the Sanctum. When this disconnect happens, we experience ourselves separate from life. We lose sight of our meaning. This makes us susceptible to losing balance as our lives often fall to pieces, and health is eroded in our experience.

The Sanctum lies beyond the shores of logical understanding, for it does not operate in the world of cause and effect. It doesn't operate in the world of space and time, and thus cannot be studied by science. It is unseen. However, it can be experienced as the soul of our being.

Exploring the Sanctum:
The Soul of the Matter

"There is no path to happiness, happiness is the path.
There is no path to love, love is the path.
There is no path to peace, peace is the path."

~ Dan Milman, from "The Way of the Peaceful Warrior"

Our Soul Purpose

The soul connects us to the Sanctum of our being from where the health creation journey arises. It is the part of ourselves that flows Vitality into our physical and psychological reality.

> Our soul purpose is not the pursuit of competing—to have more.
>
> Life already has everything …
>
> It is not a discipline of understanding through reason what life is … Life knows …
>
> It cannot be reached by trying to become better people … Life is …
>
> It cannot be grasped by studying the history of who we are … Life creates …
>
> It cannot be felt through emotional exploration or ecstasy … Life is at peace …
>
> We will not find it in our bodies—for the body is an expression of genetic inheritance gifted to us by our ancestors.

We will not find it through our senses—
there the world is reflected back to us in all
its unending diversity, colored in our own
image ...

We will not find it in our minds—for there
is a sea of perception, ideas, and beliefs,
creating our experiences.

It cannot be found in the world—for the
world is its creation.

No matter how much we look out there, we
shall not find it.

For it is looking through us.

Seeing the Sanctum

The essence of health flows from the deepest recesses of
our souls. It is a place so hard to remember, yet
impossible to forget. It is in the depths of our being, where
our soul can "see" the Sanctum of life, in the stillness of
our hearts.

In a moment of wonder we pause, and suddenly, quite
unexpectedly, we are not there anymore. As time and
space fall away, we realize in us something greater than
"I".

Aligning with this reality, we feel the Vitality of life
pulsing through us, and touch something within our
being—something that cannot be truly expressed in
words.

Having felt the Sanctum, we enter its peace and feel
the flow of Vitality as it illuminates the health creation
journey in our experience. We are simply observers now,
on a magical ride through ourselves, held safely by
something mysterious and mystical, something that lies at
the heart of life.

Even though it cannot be grasped or attained, it flows
its reality into our awareness. From the ocean of life,

Vitality fills our bodies and minds with meaning, balance, and harmony. It brings with it inspiration, insight, intuition, and experiences of serendipity that guide our lives forward. Fears and anxiety transform into confidence and well-being. Anger and pride subside into its peaceful waters.

Having found our sense of emotional freedom, our minds gravitate toward understanding and wisdom, so that we live a life that serves us, serves others, and life as a whole. We are inspired to give to the world, to love through the darkness, to create a story of inspiration and adventure through which we live our lives.

Having found our purpose and meaning we naturally act in ways to support our body and minds, focusing on our health creation rather than fighting perceptional battles that no longer serve our purpose.

As all the pieces come together—illuminating health in our own experience—our lives begin to grow through the connections we make. We feel a sense of gratitude, for we are waking up to the realization that all the treasures we have been seeking reside in our own souls ... and that we are connected to life. It is a life that knows us, loves us, and seeks to guide us towards our dreams.

This is the illumination of the Health Spectrum. As we bend our awareness through the prism of life itself, the colors fade into one. For health is one, and now we finally understand who it is we really are. We are the health we have been looking for.

Consider the Pale Blue Dot

*"Even illness becomes wellness when we replace 'I'
with a 'we'."*

~ Malcolm X

Having journeyed to the center of our own being, we can now look again at who we are. Not who we think we are, not what the world would have us believe we are, but who we are in our essence.

Health is our core identity that we not only share with every other living thing, but that which unites us to our communities, our ecosystems, and the planet as a whole.

As humanity has grown in its population and influence over the last few centuries, we have become not only the dominant species on the planet, but a species that has the capacity to do something that no other living organism has done before: to influence the health of the whole planet.

I end this chapter with one of the greatest vantage points I have ever come across, which takes a look at all of humanity. For when I speak of health in this book, I speak from the vision of a Worldwide Health. It is when we realize we all share a common identity—when we see the whole—that such a vision can come to pass. So let's take a ride far into space with the words of the late Carl Sagan, American Astronomer and Cosmologist, as he takes us on a journey into outer space to look back towards Earth, and to look at what it means to be human.

The Pale Blue Dot

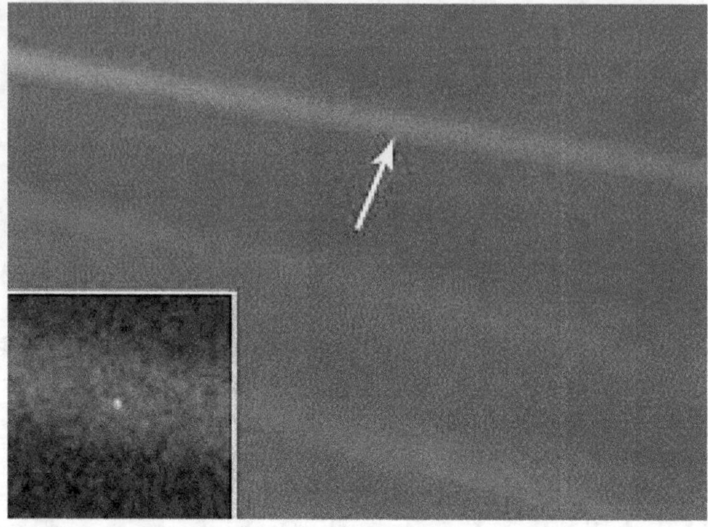

The photo above was taken by Voyager 1 in 1990 as it sailed away from Earth, more than 4 billion miles in the distance. Having completed its primary mission, Voyager at that time was on its way out of the Solar System, on a trajectory of approximately 32 degrees above the plane of the Solar System.

Ground Control issued a command that directed the distant spacecraft to turn around and, looking back, take photos of each of the planets it had visited. From Voyager's vast distance, the Earth was captured as an infinitesimal point of light (between the two white tick marks in the image), actually smaller than a single pixel of the photo.

The image was taken with a narrow angle camera lens, with the sun quite close to the field of view. Quite by accident, the Earth was captured in one of the scattered light rays, caused by taking the image at an angle so close to the sun.

Dr. Sagan was quite moved by this image of our tiny world, as he gave this reflection:

"From this distant vantage point, the Earth might not seem of any particular interest. But for us, it's different.

Consider again that dot. That's here. That's home. That's us. On it everyone you love, everyone you know, everyone you ever heard of, every human being who ever was, lived out their lives. The aggregate of our joy and suffering, thousands of confident religions, ideologies, and economic doctrines, every hunter and forager, every hero and coward, every creator and destroyer of civilization, every king and peasant, every young couple in love, every mother and father, hopeful child, inventor and explorer, every teacher of morals, every corrupt politician, every "superstar", every "supreme leader", every saint and sinner in the history of our species lived there—on a mote of dust suspended in a sunbeam.

The Earth is a very small stage in a vast cosmic arena.

Think of the rivers of blood spilled by all those generals and emperors so that in glory and triumph they could become the momentary masters of a fraction of a dot. Think of the endless cruelties visited by the inhabitants of one corner of this pixel on the scarcely distinguishable inhabitants of some other corner. How frequent their misunderstandings, how eager they are to kill one another, how fervent their hatreds. Our posturings, our imagined self-importance, the delusion that we have some privileged position in the universe, are challenged by this point of pale light.

Our planet is a lonely speck in the great enveloping cosmic dark. In our obscurity—in all this vastness—there is no hint that help will come from elsewhere to save us from ourselves.

The Earth is the only world known, so far, to harbor life. There is nowhere else, at least in the near future, to which our species could migrate. Visit, yes. Settle, not yet.

Like it or not, for the moment, the Earth is where we make our stand. It has been said that astronomy is a humbling and character-building experience. There is perhaps no better demonstration of the folly of human conceits than this distant image of our tiny world. To me, it underscores our responsibility to deal more kindly with one another and to preserve and cherish the pale blue dot, the only home we've ever known.

~ Carl Sagan, Pale Blue Dot: A Vision of the Human Future in Space, 1997 reprint.

Conclusion

"The world is waiting … anticipating."

~ Roger Hamilton, "Wink"

We have traveled a long way on our journey to discover the nature of health. We have discovered that health can be found deep within life in the Sanctum of our being. It flows outward via the field of Vitality into our physical and psychological realities. We explored the 12 principles underpinning its intelligence—the principles that form the foundation upon which life can create itself in a healthy manner. They are a core identity we share with all of life.

We have seen how this intelligence is embodied as an innate meaning that can be expressed as our unique purpose, how it balances our physical and psychological realities, and activates our creativity that sparks harmony to manifest within our relationships. These keys allow us to grow and create our lives in a healthy manner. This experience helps us realize we belong to a greater whole. We belong to all of life, where compassion, love, and peace are natural expressions of this larger reality.

We have also reflected on the the way health can be eroded in our lives. We have seen the way Perceptional Reality forms a paradigm of seeing the world that separates us, creates conflict, and makes us believe that life is founded on a polar black-and-white world, where struggle and suffering are unavoidable. We have seen how this "illusion", when expressed as a reality in our minds and bodies, erodes our health. It erodes our health, not only on the physical and psychological levels that undermine our own lives, but also on the social and environmental levels. Indeed, the fact that much of human society is still founded on Perceptional Reality drives the creation of the many social and environmental problems we now face as a human species.

Humanity, in its current level of development, has unprecedented ability to influence not only individual lives, not only lives of social groups, but of every single living life form on planet Earth.

Our technological development, our immense population growth in the last century, and our ever-increasing use of natural resources means that who we choose to be, what we choose to believe, and the way we behave, affects the health of the whole planet.

It is at this critical juncture of human evolution that we are faced with a choice. It is a choice that may well determine the destiny of the human species.

> *Will we continue down the pathways that are perceptional in nature?*
>
> *Will we continue to strive to become "bigger", "better", and "more" by destroying the natural resources that we see as things to be used to our ends without considering the way they belong to the greater whole?*
>
> *Will we not see that this approach is destroying our balance with nature, and eroding the harmony of the environmental systems of the world? It is an erosion of health that will increasingly impact humanity, creating illness in our social structures because of the interdependent relationship we have with all of life.*
>
> *Will we continue to believe that conflict and war are ways to demonstrate our strength, blinded to the fact that another world war would destroy civilization as we know it*

with the nuclear technology that we, as humans, possess?

Will we continue to hold onto outdated mythological beliefs that create a dualistic world in our perception where men and women fight gender wars, and society fractures into the rich minority and the poor majority?

Will we continue to live through perceptions that destabilize our physical and psychological health, or will we choose again, and align our reality with the way life creates itself?

Will we seek freedom in our expression, by choosing that which maintains meaning, balance, and harmony in our lives, the lives of others, and life on Earth?

It may seem that these choices are out of our hands. The forces that have created our culture are playing out without our ability to intervene, beyond our control, and above the everyday choices we make as individuals. Yet, just like gardens are made of flowers, our societies are made of individual people like you and I. The very personal choices we make as individuals ripple out to affect the whole.

"The world is waiting ... anticipating."

What will you choose?

What identity will you adapt?

Who will you become?

How will you choose to live your life?

The reason why understanding and living within the identity of health is such an important journey to undertake, is because it is the platform upon which life stands. It enables us to transcend the conflicts in our inner world, so that this can flow outwards, and create a healthy reality in our own lives.

If we do this as individuals, as a society, and as a humanity, it can become the ark that can take us safely through the floods of uncertainty and turmoil afflicting human social structures.

> *Do you have the courage to look inside? The courage to make a stand and take the Health Creation journey to discover who it is you are in your essence? To journey into yourself, face your fears, your prejudices, your pride, and your ignorance?*

Let them go, and choose an identity that does not support the perceptional pathways that are eroding health in your life.

Look deeper within and realize that underneath your perceptional scripting resides the flow of Vitality, which when embraced, has the ability to align your life with the principles of health—a shared identity that allows us to live freely and express our diversity in a way that adds to the rich tapestry of life, rather than throwing us into conflict and destroying it.

This choice does not only affect our lives, or the lives of humanity—it now affects the lives of all living things on the planet.

Health is a unified reality. We have reached a point of no return as a species. We live as a global village now and we require a breakthrough that will serve us all, or we risk destroying ourselves as a species and the natural world to which we belong.

I hope you answer "yes". I hope we all find the courage to look closely at our own shadows, with compassion. Compassion to accept ourselves as we are. To forgive ourselves and others for the mistakes we have made, and to let go of any identity that does not serve us.

I hope we instead choose an identity that has greater maturity as a species—one that is aware of the gifts of life that have been bestowed upon us as humans, and which lead to the creation of not only our physical and psychological health, but our social health, and the health of the natural world.

As this book comes to its conclusion, perhaps the most important realization is the awareness that health is already here. It is here right now, right where we are. It is here to guide us on our path.

After all, we are life, and as such, we are the magic we have been looking for ...